Gin, Ale and Poultices
... Lasers and Scanners

JOY WOODALL

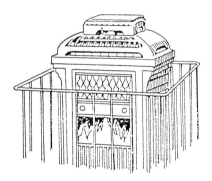

Solihull Workhouse & Hospital
1742 - 1993

ISBN 0 9504039 6 2

Cover drawn by George Busby

Plans drawn by Edna Hale

Additional drawings by George Busby and Kit Startin

Published by Joy Woodall, Solihull

Printed by Louis Drapkin Limited, Allcock Street, Birmingham B9 4EA

FOREWORD

Just over a year ago I was invited by John Clark, the General Manager, to write a short history of Solihull Workhouse and Hospital to mark the opening of the new District General Hospital. It has proved to be a most fascinating project which I have very much enjoyed. I hope the following pages will be of interest to patients and staff, past and present, and the people of Solihull in general.

The Workhouse first opened its doors to the 'undeserving poor' some 155 years ago. Subsequently those at the bottom of the social pile, both temporarily and permanently — the poor, the sick, the aged and infirm, children, 'lunatics', 'imbeciles', tramps, and those with smallpox and TB — filled its wards. Although, in time, many of these groups went to other special institutions, the Workhouse continued to be busy. Then the circumstance of war turned it into a Hospital. Now, 55 years on, a new phase is about to begin.

In 1982 I helped the late Dr Doris Quinet publish her book 'Paul Quinet'. The memory of my conversations with her about Paul, her doctor husband, and the Hospital have greatly assisted my research, as have my more recent talks with Miss Nan Freeman. Miss Freeman has given me much useful information about the Infirmary, and the Hospital, where she nursed for a time, in the first years of the war. I would also like to thank Sue Bates, Dr Denis Gray, Dr John Robson, and all those kind people who have helped by recalling their memories of the Hospital. I am especially grateful, however, to Dr Brian Gough and Mr Harold Watson without whose detailed remembrances, advice and expertise my task would have been extremely difficult; both have given most generously of their time.

For permitting the reproduction of photographs in their possession I would like to thank Sue Bates, Miss Freeman, Dr Gough, Dr Gray, Mr J. R. Pettman, Mr Watson, Aerofilms Ltd, The Birmingham Post and Mail Ltd, Solihull Libraries and Arts, The Solihull News and Solihull Hospital.

I would particularly like to thank Edna Hale for so expertly drawing the plans, and George Busby for his excellent cover. On the production side I would like to thank June Lawrence and the Picture Library of the Birmingham Post for help with photographs, Rita Bishop, David Jenkinson and last but by no means least my husband, John, who took numerous photographs for me and spent many frustrating hours at the word-processor struggling with my handwriting, spelling and punctuation.

Joy Woodall
January 1994

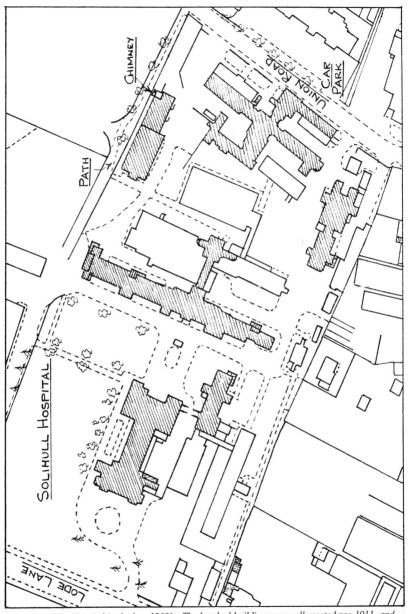

A plan of the Hospital in the late 1960's. The hatched buildings were all erected pre 1911, and the others mostly post 1940. At this time quite a large area of the grounds was still set out in lawns and flower borders.   (EH)

4

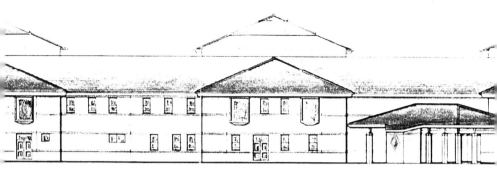

The opening of the new District General Hospital in 1994 will be an important event in Solihull's history. For the first time the people of the area will have a modern purpose-built hospital where all types of treatment, including the care of children, the elderly and the mentally ill will be provided on one site. No longer will it be necessary for patients to travel to Birmingham or other parts of the Borough for certain services. There will be new operating theatres, intensive care facilities and a 24-hour accident and emergency service.

The extended site, taking in the land between the present hospital and Grove Road, allows space for the new main building to be only two storeys high. Of brick construction with a tiled roof, it has 400 beds in 15 wards, each having a mixture of single- and multi-patient rooms; all have natural daylight and fresh air.

The new building will augment the Maternity Block, opened in 1972, the Outpatients and Pharmacy Departments, opened in 1987, and the staff accommodation, Apsley House and Physiotherapy built between 1968 and 1980. All other, older, buildings will be swept away and by 1996, when the final phase of construction is completed, Solihull will have a thoroughly modern hospital. For both staff and patients this will be the realisation of a long held dream.

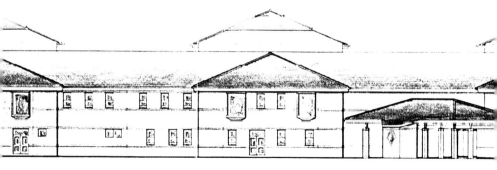

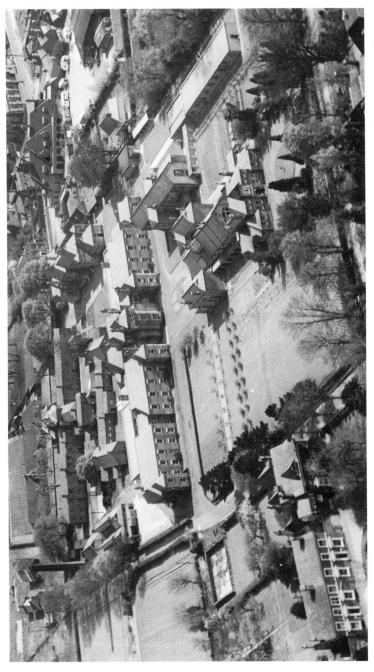

An aerial photograph of the Hospital taken on 16th April 1949. Few changes had taken place and the buildings and grounds look much as they had since 1911. In the foreground is a narrow and tree lined Lode Lane, and to the left of the Hospital drive the houses, Netherwood and Wayside, used by the Hospital. A wartime flat roofed building is on the right and two others are behind the Infirmary Block, beyond which is the oldest part of the Workhouse complex. (A)

TIME AND TENDER LOVING CARE

Until 1939 there was no hospital at Solihull. The idea of starting one — a small, cottage hospital — had first been suggested in the late 1920's or early 1930's. Numerous events were organized to raise funds including from 1932 an annual Carnival in which àll the town participated. At this time Solihull was quite rural with a population of some 25,000 but during the 1930's it started to grow, new housing springing up particularly in the Shirley area: by 1939 the population had doubled.

Compared with today, medical treatment in the 30's was quite unsophisticated but excellent work was done by local general practitioners, some of whom were surgeons, assisted by time and tender loving care. Those requiring hospital treatment went to private nursing homes, of which there were several in Solihull and Birmingham or to hospitals in Birmingham. Such treatment was not free, although some hospitals took a number of patients who were treated without charge, but these 'free beds' were not easy for Solihull residents to obtain. There was very little wholly free medical care at this time apart from 'the panel'* and many people belonged to a medical club or fund which paid out small sums when illness occurred. This rarely covered the cost of an operation which in any case most people would be very reluctant to undergo. Operations were not as routine as they are today and were considered a very serious matter. The anaesthetic then used was generally ether which could make patients very sick when they recovered consciousness, and limited the duration of any operation to a maximum of two hours. Without the benefit of modern drugs the post operative period could be painful and the convalescence slow. This frequently meant a loss of wages and sometimes a job.

Even those who could afford hospital treatment often preferred to stay in their own home and have the operation performed on a well scrubbed kitchen table, and be nursed by their own family under the doctor's supervision. Children's tonsils in particular were often removed in this way. Dr Paul Quinet, a Solihull GP and surgeon, and his wife, Dr Doris Quinet, also a GP and an anaesthetist, performed many kitchen table operations in Solihull homes often working in unsatisfactory circumstances. The folding operating table, which

*A list of doctors prepared to accept as patients people registered under the National Insurance Act.

they used in many local homes into the 1940's, still exists. With their colleague Dr E. F. Page, another local GP, they were particularly keen to see the founding of a cottage hospital where better conditions might prevail.

Preparing for War.

In 1938 war with Germany became a possibility and emergency plans were formulated. The Red Cross and St John's Ambulance Brigade, foreseeing the need for people with First Aid and nursing skills, offered classes throughout the country. A great many ladies, including those of Solihull, attended them with enthusiasm, quite a number taking up nursing professionally as a result. At the same time the Government inaugurated the Emergency Medical Service, part of its brief being to ensure that every region had sufficient hospitals and facilities for the many casualties it feared would occur should war be declared. Many Workhouses (officially Public Assistance Institutions) were considered suitable for use and requisitioned, including Solihull which in this way became an Emergency Hospital. Paul Quinet was appointed surgeon, Doris Quinet anaesthetist and Dr Eric Page (son of Dr E. F. Page) the Medical Officer (MO), having recently taken over this post at the Workhouse from his father. At the same time all three still continued in general practice. Mr Hugh Donovan, a Birmingham surgeon, was to be the Commandant of the Hospital and Mr Joe Sankey, also of Birmingham, was to assist if required. As the inmates of the Workhouse still remained Mr Horace B. Wilson, the Master, continued in his post, but in addition becoming the Hospital Secretary.

Setting up the Hospital was no easy task. Parts of the Workhouse were a hundred years old and although subsequent building had taken place all sections had always received heavy and constant use. Conditions in the Infirmary Wards (now Wards 1-4), which were to become the Hospital Wards, were primitive. Heated by large ugly coal stoves situated in the centre of the rooms, they had bare wooden floors, were badly equipped and, by hospital standards, almost impossible to keep clean. Cockroaches and steam flies were everywhere. These wards were occupied by the sick poor, many of whom were long stay, elderly, incontinent and bedridden. There were four sections on two floors, the men's wards downstairs, the women's up; there was no lift. Sister Jarret who was in charge of the Infirmary and acted as Assistant Matron did her best to care for her patients but it was an uphill task.

There was a great lack of equipment and facilities which needed to be rectified before the Workhouse could function as a Hospital. An Operating Theatre unit was created in a group of small rooms off a corridor in the Infirmary Block, the windows initially being blacked-out with hardboard although later blinds

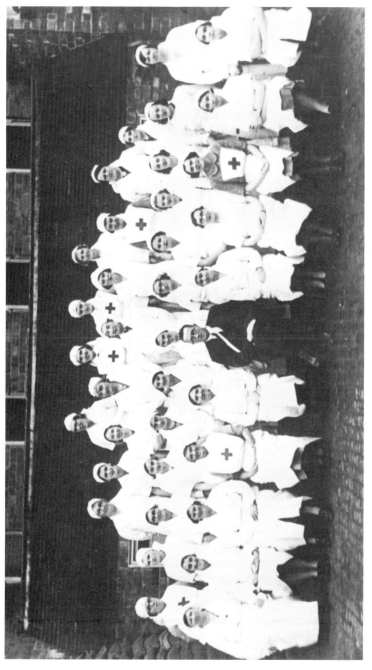

The Red Cross and Auxiliary Nurses, October 1939. Those who can be identified are, left to right:
Front Row — Sister Cook, Miss Cook, Mrs Beale, Mrs Dando, Dr Thomas, Miss Lane, Mrs Gordon-Hughes, Miss Kirby, Mrs Twiss.
Second Row — Miss Wheal, Jessie Croxton, Dorothy Croxton, Mrs Counter, Mrs Harrison-Johnson (?).
Third Row — Moira Allum, Nan Freeman, Mrs Arculus, Mrs Payne, Miss Southerton, Rene Boddington.
Back Row — Miss Southerton, Molly Raines, Mrs Lambert. (NF)

9

were obtained. They were protected on the outside by sandbags. These rooms had been used previously for the Workhouse maternity cases. There was no X-ray Department or even, to start with, an X-ray machine. On a few occasions, when an X-ray was thought essential, patients were taken to Dr Quinet's home and practice at 681 Warwick Road (now Quinet House) where he had his own machine. Here he took the X-rays and developed the film himself. Not until July 1942 was a machine acquired. Another shortage was of instruments, there not being enough to perform a fairly simple appendix-type operation. Dr Quinet had his own which he always carried with him but other surgeons had to manage as best they could. The lighting in the Operating Theatre was so inadequate that the surgeons wore battery-run headlamps, similar to miners, and at times lamps had to be handheld over the patient. Needless to say there was no Casualty Theatre, Physiotherapy or Pathology Departments, and Balkan frames, on which fractured legs were supported by ropes and pulleys, had to be made by the staff. There was even a lack of safe, clean cupboard space for dressings, medicine and drugs. A small Dispensary opened for only two hours a day. Staff was in short supply and at first the Hospital appears to have been kept going by Dr Page, Drs Paul and Doris Quinet, Matron Williams, Mary Reeves who ran the Theatre, Sister Jarret and a stalwart band of approximately 35 Red Cross and Auxiliary nurses, trained locally at the First Aid classes and now nursing professionally. Over the years the latter gained a wealth of practical experience and played a vital part in keeping the Hospital working.

These ladies when on Air Raid night duty, and in 1939 a Blitzkreig was expected, were obliged to sleep on the Hospital premises. They bedded down in the First Aid Post, on call, should a raid occur. This had previously been part of the Tramps' Block; it was dirty and flea ridden and initially they had to sleep on the floor wrapped in blankets and still be clean and fit for duty the following day.

The heavy bombing expected in the autumn of 1939 thankfully did not take place and it was mid-1940 before there were any raids and casualties in the Midland area. In October and November 1940 Birmingham and Coventry were bombarded night after night and on the night of 14th/15th November much of Coventry including the Cathedral was destroyed. By this time Solihull Hospital was more organized with extra staff and equipment.

The first resident House Surgeon, a young lady, was followed in October 1941 by Dr Harold B. Watson who was to devote the next 41 years to the Hospital, retiring in 1982. Sister Jeffcoat arrived to be Theatre Sister, Dr Brian Gough to join Mrs Quinet as an anaesthetist and Miss Windridge became Matron in place of Miss Williams. A standard Boyle anaesthetic machine was acquired and eventually the long awaited X-ray apparatus, to be followed later by a first-class Radiologist, Dr Israelski who had trained in Berlin. The much needed surgical instruments also arrived, Dr Watson obtaining these by simply ordering them direct from the suppliers (Philip Harris) the bill, for £750, being sent to Warwickshire County Council (WCC), Solihull then being under their administration. Such high-handed extravangance resulted in a personal visit from Alderman Ryland, Chairman of WCC and of the Poor Law Committee who, in time, agreed the resulting care of patients justified the unauthorised expenditure.

By Christmas 1941 the tramps, who for years had appeared at the Workhouse gate late each afternoon looking for a bed for the night, had ceased to call at Solihull. There were, however, still about 30 men who lived at the Workhouse permanently and earned their keep by working in the gardens, growing vegetables and flowers and keeping the grounds in immaculate order under the guiding eye of two professional gardeners. There were women too who filled their days by helping in the laundry. All these people had been sent there because they did not conform to society's norm: a woman with a withered arm, the profoundly deaf, the dumb, spastics, epileptics, those who had no family or anyone to care.

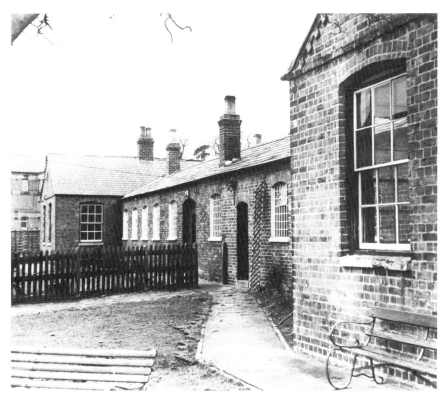

The living quarters of the female permanent inmates. *(CJ)*

One of these men, Mick, acted as porter about the Hospital. He carried the coal up to the wards for the stoves and did errands such as buying newspapers and cigarettes for the patients. The permanent inmates had separate quarters, the women living in an H-shaped single storey building in the middle of the Workhouse complex and the men on the upper floor of the Tramps' Block. They slept in dormitories taking their meals in the huge Dining Hall (now the canteen) behind the Master's House. They were cared for medically by the Hospital although they remained in the official charge of Mrs Wilson, the Workhouse Master's wife. Mr and Mrs Wilson lived on the premises in the house, now offices, facing onto Lode Lane.

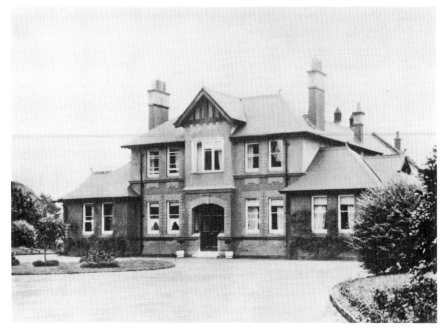

The Workhouse Master's House about 1928, now Administration. (SB)

There were also 65 long-stay chronic sick people being cared for, although they had been moved into another building, now Wards 6 and 7, so that the old Infirmary Wards might be given over entirely to the Hospital patients. An Outpatients Department was started on the ground floor at the balcony end of the Main Block (Wards 1-4) but after the tramps ceased to call, it was transferred to the ground floor of the Tramps' Block. This was already divided into cubicles and had wash rooms where the tramps had been obliged to bath before admittance. In addition a Gynaecological and Obstetrics Department was begun, this being Dr Watson's special interest and was housed upstairs at the balcony end of the Main Block; the ground floor then being given over to Orthopaedics.

By the Spring of 1942 the WCC had purchased the large house in Lode Lane next to the Hospital drive, and also the three pairs of semi-detached houses adjoining it. The large house, Wayside, became a Nurses Home; the first pair of houses — Netherwood — became a maternity unit and the others — Apsley and Ardenne — provided much improved accommodation for those who society had cast out. Later another house, across Lode Lane, was acquired providing further accommodation for these people.

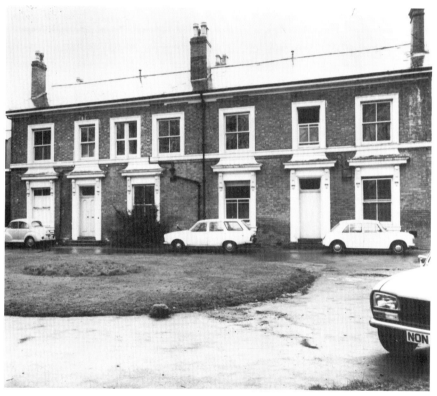

Netherwood, two Victorian houses used as a maternity unit from 1942-1972 and demolished 1978. (Courtesy Solihull News)

On 27th July 1942 at 6.30 in the morning a German plane attempted to bomb the Solihull Gas Works off Moat Lane. Instead, houses in Alston Road and Cornyx Lane were hit and demolished or badly damaged. People were still in bed or just getting up; 26 were killed, including one whole family, and many seriously injured. This was the Hospital's busiest and most testing time. Drs Quinet and Watson dealt with the surgical cases, Miss Windridge and her nurses working throughout the day in the Theatre and wards to make the injured comfortable. At 6p.m. the Hospital Commandant and Professor Seymour Barling of Birmingham arrived to see how everyone was coping. They were delighted to find that the crisis was over and that all concerned had been treated. The Hospital had been tried and not found wanting. Consequently patient numbers and the work load grew as local GP's used the Hospital more, confident of its ability.

By 1944 Dr Watson, now Resident Surgical Officer, Medical Superintendent and Obstetrics Registrar, had set up with Dr Wilfred Gaisford paediatric and neo-natal clinics at the maternity unit where Professor Beckwith Whitehouse and Mr Barnie Adshead came to advise on special cases. At Netherwood a premature baby unit was created; it had two cots in an air-conditioned room, a new and revolutionary idea. Here the Hospital achieved a remarkable success.

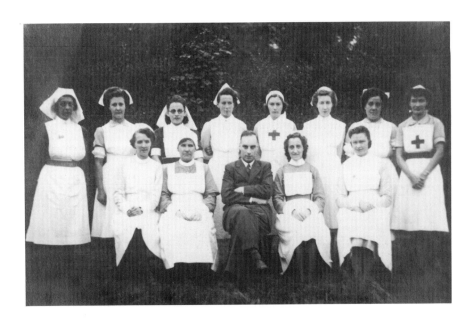

*The Netherwood **Maternity staff with Dr Harold Watson** in 1943.*
Seated next to him, right, is the sister in charge. **(HBW)**

A lady who had previously lost several babies towards the end of pregnancy through rhesus incompatibility of blood group was admitted and observed carefully. Blood grouping was only recently understood and techniques for dealing with incompatibility were not fully developed. When in the eighth month the baby began to show signs of distress, a Caesarian section was performed and a crude method of exchanging the baby's blood performed by Dr Gaisford. The baby was then placed in the premature unit where it survived. This achievement was well written up in Medical journals and Solihull maternity unit obtained great respect and as a result a number of similar cases were undertaken. Dr Watson also ran ante-natal clinics at Rugby and Nuneaton and did general surgery at Solihull with Dr Quinet.

From the time the Hospital started, fitting all the departments and the Workhouse inmates into the available buildings was a problem. When a full-time Dispensary was set up it was placed on the ground floor of a wing in the oldest part of the Workhouse. For years the department struggled to work in these cramped and decrepit conditions, the building having been condemned as unfit before the war. The acquisition of the houses in Lode Lane helped to relieve some of the congestion and when, in 1943/44, the Emergency Medical Service permitted the building of a new Operating Theatre, Plaster Room and X-ray Room adjoining the original Theatre, conditions were much improved. At the same time, elsewhere in the grounds, two new single storey wards, numbers 5 and 8, were erected. More wards were needed as some patients remained in hospital for months occupying beds which now, with modern techniques, would be vacated within days. In 1945 a young girl with a broken thigh was in Ward 1 for more than three months; her leg was supported by a Balkan frame for at least nine weeks and she had not set her foot to the ground after 11 weeks. Nowadays she would be home within three weeks.

When the war ended in May 1945 the future of the Hospital became uncertain, a reoccurring prospect until 1972. The staff, and particularly Dr Quinet, were greatly opposed to its closure, the authorities however were doubtful about the conditions overall. But Solihull did need its Hospital: the Rover Car Company and several small industrial firms which had come to the town during the war wanted to remain; there were plans at Government level for Solihull to grow, and this would lead, in time, to a huge rise in the population; in addition the National Health Act, passed in 1946, promised that from 1948 there would be free health care. As plans for the Health Service were formulated Solihull Hospital was included being expected to provide medical care for the local area in the coming years.

There were changes in staff, new people came, including a group of recently demobilized young men who joined the Hospital as theatre orderlies. They included Reg Price who later joined the Ambulance Service, Joe Harris who became Theatre Technician and Bill Laxton later a senior nurse; each gave in the region of 30 years service to the Hospital.

The start of the National Health Service on 5th July 1948 made free health care available to all who wanted it: young and old, rich and poor. The idea of offering every man, woman and child birth to grave treatment when they were ill, including the care of eyes and teeth plus all medicines without charge was revolutionary; an ambitious experiment watched critically by countries all over the world.

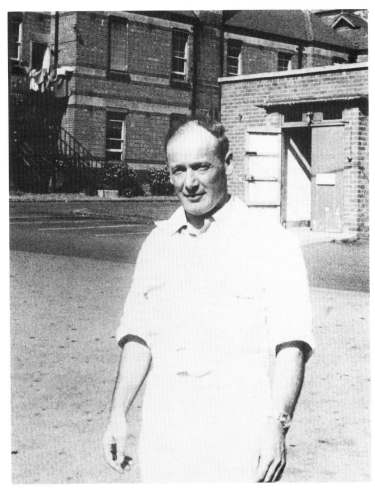

Joe Harris, the Theatre Technician, in 1957.   (HBW)

'. . . WHILE NATURE CURES THE DISEASE'

For many centuries those who were sick had to rely for their care and treatment upon their family, friends and neighbours. Only the wealthy could afford a qualified doctor, which was probably just as well, for the treatments prescribed usually involved bleeding, purging and fasting which often did more harm than good. In fact there was little anyone could do for the sick but relieve symptoms, suppress pain, and wait for nature to effect a cure. Most housewives had old family recipes from which to make simple remedies and invariably there was a local wise woman who, understanding the healing properties of herbs and plants, might be consulted in serious cases. If the illness was really bad someone would go to the nearest town where there was usually an apothecary who sold drugs, spices and herbs, and made up medicines and compounds which might contain weird and exotic ingredients; he also acted as a doctor to the poor.

Illness often led to hardship and, not invariably, to poverty but since Elizabeth I's great Poor Law Act of 1601 the poor had been helped, in some measure, by parish relief: the payment of money and/or goods to those in need. Administered by each parish the relief was paid out of a compulsory levy to which all the parishioners subscribed according to their holding of land.

In the late 17th century the divisions in society grew, it became less neighbourly and caring; increasingly men and women who had illness in their home had to ask for help from the parish. The earliest surviving references to people in Solihull being relieved due to sickness date from 1658.

> 16 Nov   Gave Richard Brick & John Swinford being sick   1/- each
> Widow Grant almost blind   1/-
> Richard Veales haveing beene long sick   1/-
> Rich Cottrell beene long sicke   6d

At this time Solihull was a small decayed market town. There was no doctor but one, John Short, possibly an apothecary, attempted cures.

> 3rd July   John Short for letting Wid Durhams blood in her foote to help her lamenesse   4d
> 10th Dec   Pd John Short at severall tymes for care of William Wilcoxe hand by consent of the parish   £2.0.0

Short was still busy in 1671 when he was paid 'for a cure done upon Mary Burch 10/-'.

During the 18th century there was considerable development in medicine nationally, the number of doctors increased and medical practise improved. Hospitals for the sick poor were founded in London and inoculation against smallpox was taken up enthusiastically by the rich. By the late 1730's the cost of caring for the sick poor in Solihull had increased considerably: a Doctor Miles was paid for attending numerous paupers and for drugs which he prescribed; some poor people were paid to 'nurse' others who were ill and the parish occasionally paid for midwives and support during 'lying in'.

The Parish Workhouse

One of the basic tenets of the Poor Law was that everyone capable of working should do so and if they could not find work themselves it would be provided by the parish. Gradually the idea of a special building, a work house, where the poor could live and work together under proper supervision, grew up. The first work house was built in Bristol in 1696 and others soon followed. The results were considered excellent and in 1723 an Act of Parliament permitted

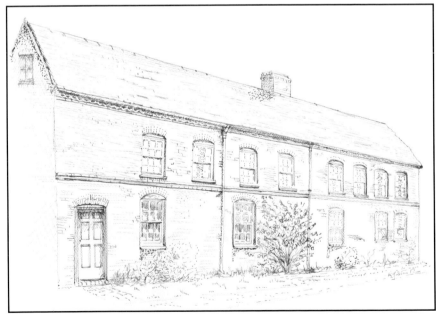

Conjectural drawing of how the Parish Workhouse may have looked in the late 18th century.   (Drawn by Kit Startin)

any parish, with the consent of the inhabitants, to acquire a building suitable for a workhouse. Those who refused to enter when sent there were deprived of any further assistance. At a public meeting in April 1740, the people of Solihull decided that a workhouse was needed, the annual cost of relieving the sick and poor having risen from £84 in 1692 to £230 in 1739.

The parish officers found a house to rent and a levy of 6d (2½p) in the pound was raised to convert it, but the building needed considerable repair and they determined to build new instead. Thomas Sandal, the builder, erected a two storey brick building with attics on the north side of Warwick Road; it still exists today and is now offices. It had a kitchen, brewhouse, pantry, long room, store room, two cellars, two chambers over the kitchen, a chamber over the long room, infirmary, garret and long room garret.

The first Master, Joseph Hammond, was engaged in December 1742 at a salary of £25 per annum. The inmates worked and lived together in the long room furnished with tables, chairs, forms and three spinning wheels. Some spun whilst the rest ran the house by cooking, cleaning, washing, gardening and brewing. There were 20 beds upstairs although by 1773, when 22 people entered the Workhouse, there were only 12 mattresses and 17 bedsteads. By this date the inmates were busy carding and spinning woollen and linen yarn and making shoes perhaps for sale or for the use of the poor.

From 1796 the able-bodied poor were no longer forced into workhouses and from this time the occupants were chiefly those too young, too ill or too old to work. In the early 1800's there were between 30 and 50 paupers in Solihull Workhouse — some children, at least 13 women and about 20 men — some of them very old. The men kept pigs and grew turnips, cabbages, potatoes, peas and beans. The women spun both wool and flax for which they were paid, the rate being 1d to 1½d (less than ½p) for spinning a lea (300 yards) of flax. In 1804 the payment was cut and a number took up dress and bonnet making instead.

The food was purchased from local tradesmen, the main regular items being milk, meat, cheese and salt although oatmeal, malt, hops, butter, lard, tea, sugar, treacle, vinegar and black pepper were bought occasionally. Delivered on Wednesday and Saturday at 10 a.m., the goods were weighed by the Master to ensure they were correct; bills were paid quarterly. In 1803-5 13½ tons of coal were used in 16 months to heat the Workhouse, the cost being £11.6.1½ (£11.30½p). For the sick the only panacea was alcohol, '1 pint of cowslip wine 8d' 'A ¼ of Gin 5d' and '1 pint of Ale 3d' being purchased, and occasionally, white bread 'for Poultices'.

The national population, rising since about 1760, continued to increase and the burden on the ratepayers of supporting the poor and needy and their large families, both in and out of the workhouses, grew. It became so great that the whole system creaked and was in danger of breaking down. Consequently a new Act was passed in 1834, completely reforming the system. The parishes were grouped into Unions administered by a Board of Guardians and controlled by Commissioners in London, although the ratepayers still provided the funds.

The Union Workhouse —
'A brick and mortar elysium'!

The Solihull Union included 11 parishes — Knowle, Temple Balsall, Baddesley Clinton, Packwood, Lapworth, Nuthurst, Barston, Elmdon, Tanworth, Yardley, Solihull — the three latter each having a workhouse. The Guardians decided that none were suitable; they would buy land and build a new Union Workhouse, capable of holding 125 paupers. In August 1837 Mr James B. Harper of Henley-in-Arden was engaged to erect the new Workhouse, Solihull having been chosen

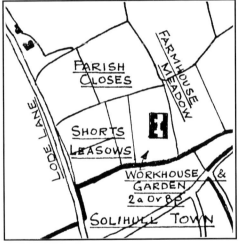

as the most suitable place for it. A field situated just off Warwick road, 2 acres 0 roods 8 perches in size, was purchased from Rev Archer Clive, the rector of Solihull and also a Guardian, for £236. The Guardians paid all the expenses including fencing, ditching etc. and making a roadway at least 20 feet wide to give access to the fields beyond. A loan of £3,500 was arranged and work began.

The access, now Union road, ran in front of the new Workhouse which consisted of two long buildings parallel to each other and joined by a central block and tower. The final cost was

Sketch plan, based on the Tithe Map c1840, of the Union Workhouse area.   (EH)

£4,248.17.11 (£4,248.89½p), including the land and furnishings. The post of Workhouse Master and Matron was advertised in January 1838, at a joint salary of £70 per annum. Job Genders and his wife were appointed and took up their duties immediately at the old Workhouse. On 12th September 1838 the paupers were moved to the new Union Workhouse 'heated by Hot Water Apparatus' to start life under the new regime. The old building passed into the hands of the Solihull Charity Estate and was converted into three houses.

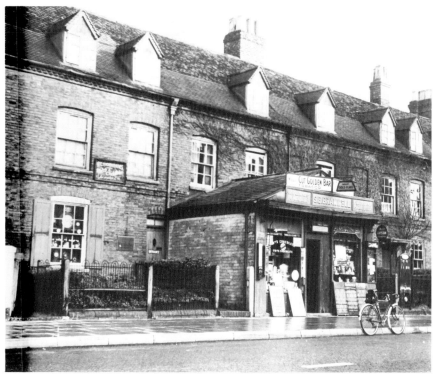

The old Parish Workhouse in the late 1940's,
about a century after it was converted into houses.   (DG)

The basic intention of the 1834 Act was to abolish out-relief to the able-bodied poor. Except for occasional illness and for apprenticing their children they were to receive help only if they entered the workhouse. Once inside life was not meant to be pleasant, aiming to make them wish to leave as soon as possible and live 'by their own honest industry'. To this end conditions in the workhouse were to be less attractive than the worst possible life beyond its walls, including the diet, designed to be just at subsistence level and very dull. Breakfast each day was 6oz bread (5oz women) and 1½ pints gruel. Dinner three days per week was 5oz cooked meat and ½lb potatoes; three days 1½ pints soup and on Friday 14oz suet or rice pudding (12oz women). Supper four nights a week was 6oz bread (5oz women) with 2oz cheese and three nights 6oz bread (5oz women) with 1½ pints broth. Children under nine years had a special diet and those over nine the same as the women. Old people over 60 might have 1oz tea, 5oz butter and 7oz sugar per week for breakfast instead of gruel, if it was expedient.

This better breakfast for the elderly reflected the Poor Law Commissioners concern for the sick, aged and infirm who were to be treated 'with marked tenderness and care' and, where possible, were to remain in the community and receive out-relief. Those who did enter a workhouse were to be offered 'distinct, quiet and comfortable abodes'. But the Solihull Guardians did not exactly follow these rules and the majority of the inmates of the Solihull Union were the aged, infirm, sick, orphans and the feeble-minded, indeed the same type of people who had inhabited the old Parish Workhouse. The able-bodied poor, by contrast, formed a minority of the total Workhouse population the number depending very much on the seasons; falling in spring, rising in autumn and particularly in very wet periods.

The inmates were under the medical supervision of Dr Thomas Lowe who practised from The Limes in Warwick Road (now Quinet House) the home of Solihull doctors from 1761-1976. He was appointed in March 1839 at a salary of £20 per annum. There was already a nurse, Mrs Jane Martin, appointed at a salary of £5 per annum and her keep.

On admittance the poor were placed in a receiving ward until they had been bathed, medically inspected and given regulation clothes to wear. Then they were segregated according to sex, age and health into seven categories, each with their own dormitory, dayroom and yard. There was a separate ward for vagrants. Except for children under seven years who could see their mothers 'at all reasonable times' and boys and girls aged 7-15 years who might meet their parents at 'one time each day', the categories were not allowed to communicate with each other. All men and women over 15 years lived apart, including married couples, although sometimes aged married couples were allowed a separate sleeping apartment. Yet at Solihull, family and friends could visit daily, at least for the first few years, quite contrary to Poor Law regulations.

The Workhouse day began at 5.45a.m., Breakfast was at 6.30-7.00a.m., Dinner at 12 noon-1p.m., Supper at 6-7p.m., Recreation at 7-8p.m. when it was bedtime. In winter the day started an hour later. The time between was occupied by work: the women and girls did all the housework and assisted the nurse with the young and infirm. They also washed and mended the sheets, which were changed once a month, and the linen and stockings of the inmates which were changed once a week. The able-bodied men were meant to work for 10 hours each day to prepare them for future employment but the task found for them, picking oakum — plucking twisted lengths of rope into fibres for caulking boats — whilst uncongenial was neither arduous nor physically demanding. The supplies of rope were intermittent and the work can hardly have fully occupied them. Some probably worked in the garden growing the quantities of potatoes consumed. The whole day, including the work and food, was dull, depressing and boring. Smoking was forbidden as were cards, dice, games of chance, writing paper and 'printed paper of an improper tendency'.

As pauperism was believed to be hereditary the Workhouse children were educated to rise above it. In 1838 a Mrs Tomlinson was appointed schoolmistress, she was followed by Matilda Holdbrook engaged in 1841 at £20 per year 'to teach and reside in the House and have the care of the children'. For at least three hours each day they were to learn reading, writing, arithmetic and the principles of the Christian religion. From 1851 only qualified teachers were employed ensuring a reasonable standard of education. The pupils had plenty of outdoor exercise, the older boys working in the garden for two afternoons a week, if they wished. The Guardians were enlightened enough to send several handicapped children to special schools for the deaf, dumb or blind where the fees might be £20 per annum. Workhouse life however was very insular, the children's only escape being the Sunday School Christmas dinner. Then from 1862 they attended the village school and thus saw more of the outside world. From the age of 11 onwards most were apprenticed or went into service although a few were sent to 'industrial schools' where they were trained for 'suitable situations'.

A Christian way of life was considered to be most important. A chaplain was appointed in 1838 at £30 per annum to oversee the moral and religious conduct of the inmates, visit the sick, teach the children, preach every Friday and administer the Sacrament to those unable to go to church. The high salary paid for his part-time work reflects the major role moral rectitude was thought to play in lifting the residents out of the Workhouse towards a better life.

In charge of all was the Workhouse Master. He was responsible for every facet of the Houses's life: admitting the paupers, enforcing industry, order, punctuality and cleanliness, reading prayers twice a day, taking roll-call. He supervised the catering and schooling, kept the accounts and a Master's Journal and reported to the Guardians on their weekly visits. Job Genders kept pigs and poultry on his own account, but this was against the rules and he had to stop. He was also reprimanded for taking improper liberties with some female paupers and threatened with dismissal if it occured again. The Matron acted as the Master's deputy and was responsible for the women and children, clothing, laundry, nursing and the female staff. At 9p.m. they visited each ward to ensure everyone was in bed and that fires and lights were out. The gates were then locked until 6a.m. next day.

In the first 10 years the Union Workhouse had an average population of between 82 and 126 people approximately half being Solihull parishioners. By 1841 51 inmates had died, 46 of them being over 50 or under 20 and all ill or 'decayed'.

Because of the number of aged and sick inmates the Guardians soon realized that the Infirmary wards were inadequate and plans were drawn up in 1840 for them to be enlarged. When completed they were equipped with 16 wooden beds and 48 blankets. The receiving wards were also too small; they were enlarged and 'more completely separated from the rest of the House'.

Dr Lowe, the Medical Officer (MO), was supposed to inspect each new inmate but he rarely attended in person. He visited so infrequently that in 1847 the patients complained of being neglected. He resigned in 1869 after 31 years service, his successor being Dr Edward Sutton Page, who was urged to visit at least twice a week. The MO's salary was now £35 per annum but Page like Lowe was expected to provide all medicines and surgical instruments. When the doctor was absent the Workhouse nurse was in charge. Unable to cope alone, she was assisted by female inmates who were often unsuitable and elderly. In 1872 the Infirmary still had only one trained nurse who cared for six wards. The strain often proved too much and several left and a few, such as Mrs Wood in 1874, were dismissed for being drunk on duty. The first qualified nurse with three years hospital training was Ellen Portner appointed in 1879, but a second nurse was not engaged until 1894 and only then because 35 patients, 16 of whom were bedridden, was thought to be too much for one.

The first Public Health Act was passed in 1848 as a result of the terrible cholera outbreaks which killed thousands of people living in ill-drained industrial areas; gradually many improvements took place. Solihull was a healthy place but fever cases occurred occasionally and because, of the lack of isolation facilities, were, from about 1846, placed in a converted tool-shed in the Workhouse garden. It was still in use in 1872 when an outbreak of smallpox caused the Guardians to engage a temporary nurse, but only for 10 days. The next year the Solihull Rural Sanitary Authority (RSA) was formed to look after public health locally. Dr Page had complained for some years about the inadequate isolation shed and this was now backed by others. Cases of smallpox and typhoid in 1874 and 1875 which resulted in all patients, pauper and private being nursed in the shed brought matters to a head. The RSA bought two acres of land in Wagon Lane, Olton for £405 where a proper isolation hospital, for all classes, could be set up. Opened in 1877 at a cost of £2,045 it held 12 patients, had a resident Master and Matron and a special ambulance. Initially Dr Page was MO but was soon succeeded by Dr E. H. Hardwicke. The charge per person was £2.2.0 plus £3.3.0 to the MO; in the first three years it dealt with 50 cases.

Overcrowding in the Workhouse Infirmary was a persistent problem; and in 1869 additions costing £450 were made to the male wards giving 14 extra beds. At the same time, in an unusual burst of generosity, the Guardians decided that all wards should be fitted with personal lockers giving the inmates, for the first time, somewhere to keep their few possessions. The Workhouse population of 97 in 1851 fell in 1861 to 56, but by 1871 it was 92, and 113 in 1881. When, in 1894, Dr Page complained that every ward was full, the Guardians hardly

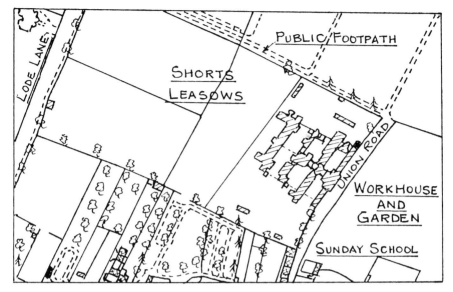

*Plan of the Union Workhouse buildings
and surrounding area about 1886.   (EH)*

responded but by way of consolation provided coco-matting for the female bathrooms and a bath-chair. The following year he demanded new isolation wards, for the Olton Hospital was often full and some smallpox and fever patients were being admitted to the Workhouse. Plans were drawn up and approved, but nothing happened. The Visiting Committee suggested the best economy, instead of piecemeal additions, was a completely new Workhouse for 320 inmates and 87 vagrants; the cost £40,641. Surprisingly, the Guardians who were always aware of the ratepayers' pockets, were very keen but gradually their enthusiasm waned and they started to cut the plans to save money. A death from diphtheria in 1898 caused the long suffering Dr Page to threaten to appeal to a higher authority if proper isolation wards were not provided, plus more room for the excess inmates. A temporary building was suggested but shelved and the lunatic ward used instead. There was much sickness and the nurses found it hard to cope but the Guardians insisted the House was not overcrowded. They did, however decide to build a new Infirmary including isolation and lying-in wards to accommodate 64 patients and new wards to house 68 tramps, the whole to cost £12,000.

'In want and misery'

The really destitute, the vagrants or tramps, were in a class of their own. The Poor Law stipulated that they were to have food and shelter but at first the Solihull Guardians made no provision for them. In the early 1860's the few tramps calling at Solihull were housed in the fever sheds, given 6oz bread for supper and for breakfast and obliged to pick oakum before leaving. By 1867 the number had grown to a weekly average of 67 tramps, in 1868 it was 99 and in 1869 149 per week. Officially they now had to give their names, be searched and bathed (but Solihull had no facilities) and work at breaking stone but this was probably not enforced. The wards where the vagrants were eventually lodged were enlarged in 1878 for £143, and again in 1884 (£650) when the Casual Act required that the tramps stay two nights and work two days. In January 1893 a tramp was found to have smallpox and the local people, worried about the health hazard of so many unkempt men, demanded that they be prevented from entering the town pubs and loitering in Warwick Road whilst waiting for the Workhouse gates to be opened. A crisis was reached in January 1894 when 350 tramps were admitted in a fortnight. After discussions Solihull appointed a 'Taskmaster' who was paid £20 per annum and working from 5.30a.m. to 10p.m. ensured the tramps laboured hard. Soon the numbers calling fell by two-thirds, even so further extensions to the Tramps' Wards were made in 1894, £1,000 being spent. It was just as well: finding sufficient manual labour to keep even the reduced numbers fully occupied was impossible. By December 1895 admissions were up again, 260 vagrants being accommodated in one week. The extra wards, planned in 1898, were very much needed; they were not opened until 1902 but from then until 1941 were occupied by successive generations of tramps.

New Buildings and Beginnings.

Until 1898 all the Workhouse buildings lay within the bounds of the two acres purchased in 1837, which were very crowded. At some point the land adjoining — three fields known as Short's Leasows measuring together 4 acres 3 roods 24 perches, previously part of the Glebe — was acquired by the Guardians for the Workhouse. The new Infirmary, a long symmetrical two-storey building of red brick cross-banded with black brick and cream stone, was erected on the field nearest the Workhouse. Well built, probably by Bragg Bros, and finely finished with decorated finials, it faced towards Lode Lane to which it was

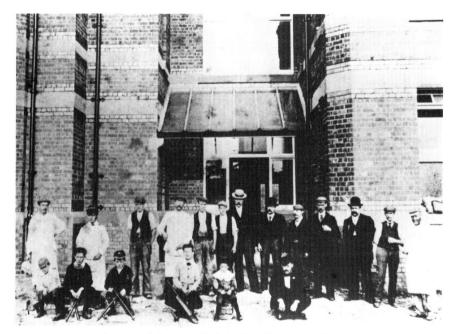

A group of the men who helped build the new Infirmary
stand outside the front entrance about 1900. (SL)

joined by a central footpath, the vehicle entrance being off Union road. The brick and stonework of the new Tramps' Block matched the Infirmary exactly but it was built beside the Workhouse within the original boundary. When opened the Tramps' Wards had to be used immediately for smallpox patients, there being a local outbreak; not until it was over were the tramps admitted.

In 1894 the RSA was swept away and replaced by Solihull Rural District Council (RDC). Yardley, growing rapidly, broke away and formed its own District Council but continued to use the Isolation Hospital at Olton almost to the exclusion of the RDC patients. A smallpox wing for 10 patients had been added in 1893 but the whole Hospital was frequently full, there being several outbreaks of scarlet fever and diphtheria at the end of the century. Meriden, which had been refused permission to send patients to Olton, suggested that a separate smallpox hospital should be built and in 1902, jointly with Solihull, bought land near Marston Green Station for £120. Ready for use in 1904 the Hospital took 16 patients, Dr Adolphus V. Bernays of Solihull, who had succeeded Dr Hardwicke at Olton, being the MO. Solihull also joined with Meriden to build a general isolation hospital leaving Olton entirely to Yardley's use. Land was purchased in Henwood Lane, Catherine de Barnes for £975 in

1907; the Hospital opened in 1910, the building having cost £8,156. The following year Yardley parish was absorbed by Birmingham and the Olton Hospital was closed.

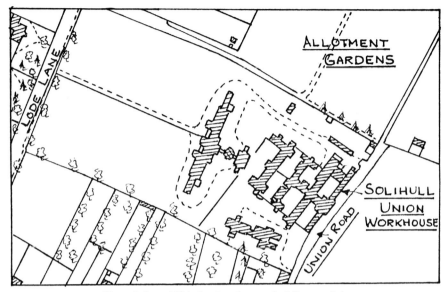

Plan of about 1904 showing the new buildings and the changes made since 1886. (EH)

Marston Green Hospital relieved the Workhouse of smallpox cases but there were many occasions prior to Catherine de Barnes Hospital opening when the isolation wards at the Workhouse were crowded. An epidemic of diphtheria and scarlet fever in February 1910 led to some children being '2 and 3 in a bed'. As a result diphtheria admissions were stopped and some patients moved from the Workhouse to Marston Green where they made good progress, although some showed signs of scarlet fever. Equally some of the 13 fever patients left in the Workhouse also showed signs of cross-infection. So serious was the outbreak that the Workhouse children were forbidden to go to school for a month and all visiting was stopped. Cross-infection was a problem elsewhere in the Infirmary, some nurses not being fully aware of the need to keep themselves, their clothes and the dressings free of infection when moving between surgical and septic cases and the maternity ward. There seems to have been a continual shortage of surgical appliances and even clothes which cannot have helped the standards of hygiene.

The new buildings seem to have given the Workhouse a new lease of life. A Ladies Visiting Committee, formed in 1895, also had an effect for they pressed for small changes which greatly improved the inmates lives. The seriously mentally ill had been long removed to the County Lunatic Asylum at Hatton but the male and female imbeciles who remained were, from 1896 at the Ladies suggestion, taken out for short walks each week. They arranged for them to have proper bathrooms, for the female lavatories to have doors, for the ambulant women patients in the Infirmary to take daily exercise in the garden, and for the Sunday exercise time for all to be increased to three hours.

From c1895 orphaned infants could be adopted and after 1902 'idiot' children were sent to Knowle Institution, now Middlefield. It was acknowledged that children should not live in the Workhouse and in 1904 a house, The Woodlands, in Friday Lane, Hampton in Arden, was rented by the Guardians as a home for 12 girls and a foster mother. Two years later a similar home for 12 boys was set up.

A novel event in 1902 was the installation of a telephone and later another in the Master's House. The next year plans to turn the old Tramps' Wards into a receiving ward, clothes store, bathroom and offices; to replan the kitchen block; make new committee and ironing rooms and convert the old Infirmary into a chapel for 125 people were soon subjected to the usual financial pruning.

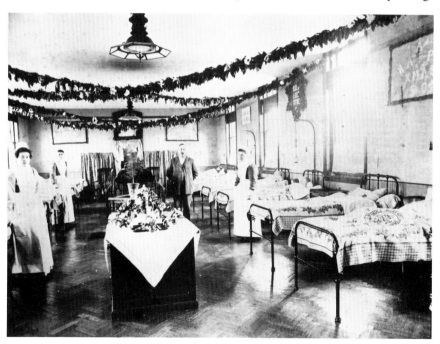

Christmas Day in the Workhouse Infirmary 1902.
The Master, W. H. Carr, and three nurses pose with patients
in a festively decorated ward. (BG)

29

The Tramps' Wards cost was reduced from £624 to £194 and the chapel plan dropped. Instead a new power laundry (£4,765) and cottage homes for the children (£2,885) were to be built. In the end the latter was abandoned in favour of The Woodlands and a laundry costing only £2,000 was completed in 1907, but there was still a need for office room and wards and a place for consumptive patients. When an administrative block with Master's House was commissioned, the idea of the chapel was again abandoned, the Dining Hall being designed to serve this purpose too. A year later ward accommodation was added to the scheme, part being intended for the chronic sick. The new Master's House, placed symmetrically between Lode Lane and the Infirmary on the two remaining fields, was a two-storey brick building with matching single-storey side wings, incorporating office space and staff bedrooms. The upper floor was pebble-dashed, with decoration in the gable and round some windows. Attached behind was the dining hall-cum-chapel and kitchen quarters. Joined to the kitchen area by a screening brick arch was a two-storey ward block. A new vehicle entrance

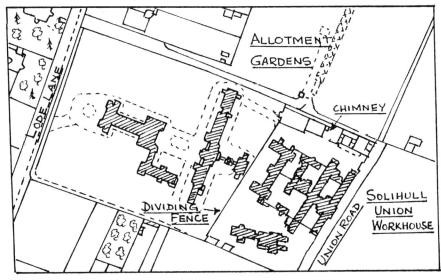

Plan of 1917 showing the buildings completed in 1910. (EH)

was made from Lode Lane to the new buildings and the Infirmary and a fence erected to divide them from the Workhouse complex. Probably at this same time the north end of the Infirmary wing was extended and finished with an ornamental iron balcony. The buildings were completed in 1910 but in 1911 the entire Workhouse was again overcrowded, inmates even being housed in the Committee Rooms. By 1912, when Dr Page had been succeeded as MO by his son, Edward F. Page, there were 200 inmates but by 1921 this had risen to 322.

The fear of being sent to the Workhouse through sick poverty caused many people to join Friendly Societies and Medical Clubs. By paying about 1½d per week a family was entitled to medicine and medical attendance when needed. Then from 1911 compulsory National Insurance for all manual workers and for all non-manual workers earning less than the income tax threshold (£160 in 1911 raised progressively to £250 in 1920 and £420 in 1942) provided the employed working class with medical treatment (the panel) and benefits during illness. Even so it left out the non-working wives and children of the insured, the unemployed and those in non-manual occupations. They could get free medical care through the Relieving Officer, which involved a means test. Free hospital care meant entering the Workhouse Infirmary and many preferred to suffer in silence rather than enter its doors. However a series of Public Health Acts improved general standards of cleanliness, of the treatment of tuberculosis, of school children's health, of midwifery, maternity and child welfare. Most babies were still born at home but the provision of a District Nurse and the Infant's Welfare Centre in the Warwick Road assisted many mothers.

In 1926 the Solihull Board of Guardians, as throughout the country, was abolished and the Workhouse passed into the control of Warwickshire County Council. The children, the mentally ill, those with TB and other notifiable diseases were cared for elsewhere but many remained. Life in Solihull Workhouse could never have been enjoyable, it was probably very dull and boring but it appears not to have been harsh or cruel. The Guardians were indecisive and cheese-paring but in the circumstances of their time they probably did their best for those in their care.

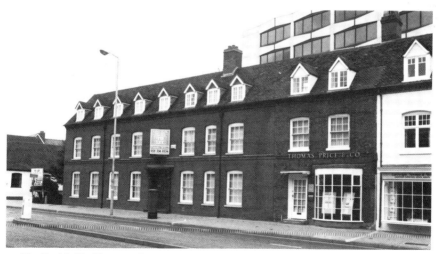

The Parish Workhouse today after considerable restoration, and road widening.   (JW)

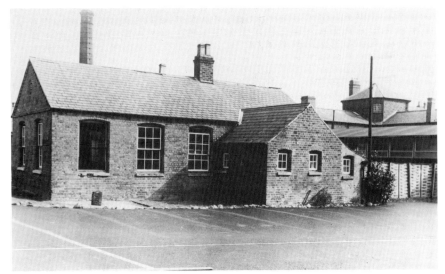

Part of the permanent inmates accommodation with the laundry chimney behind and the Workhouse tower, from which the Master could oversee the whole complex, on the right.   (CJ)

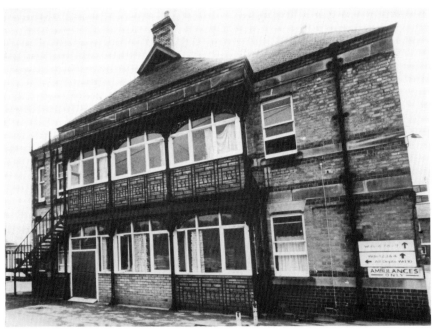

The wrought iron balcony at the north end of the Infirmary, probably added in 1910.   (SH)

UNDER THE NATIONAL HEALTH SERVICE — THE FIRST TEN YEARS

When the National Health Service started in 1948 the Ministry of Health set up 14 Regional Hospital Boards, each divided for day to day administration into local Hospital Management Committees. Solihull Hospital together with seven others — Selly Oak, Sorrento, Lordswood, Moseley Hall, Little Bromwich, The Accident and Royal Orthopaedic Hospitals — fell under the direction of the Birmingham (Selly Oak) Hospital Management Committee (BSOHMC) who controlled the spending. At Solihull there were several internal Hospital committees whose members included doctors, local councillors, the Hospital Secretary, the matron and laymen. They managed the Hospital, appointed staff, oversaw the welfare and treatment of patients and the upkeep of the buildings although almost everything had to be approved by the BSOHMC, especially financial matters or changes to the fabric.

Also under Solihull Hospital control were a number of homes and hospitals previously run by other organisations and authorities. Opposite the Hospital in Lode Lane, was Brook House opened as a Maternity Home in the 1930's by the District Nursing Infant Welfare Association and used by local GP's for patients who did not wish to have their babies at home and could afford to pay. Absorbed by the Hospital in 1949 it continued to be used by GP's who wished to attend personally at births, and supervise their patient's subsequent stay in hospital which at that time was about three weeks. The Hospital also acquired the Isolation Hospital at Catherine de Barnes, shortly to be transformed into another maternity unit, plus two other properties, The Beeches, Widney Manor Road and Eastcote Grange at Barston. The former had previously been Evans Convalescent Home for children whilst the latter, a large Victorian residence set in extensive grounds, had been used during the war by The Midland Hospital for Homoeopathic and General Treatment after being bombed out in Birmingham.

It took some time for everyone to get used to the new system but by 1951 Solihull Hospital had settled into a regular routine under a team of dedicated senior doctors, many of whom had been there for several years: Mr Quinet, since 1948 a consultant surgeon; Mr Watson the Hospital Superintendent and Gynaecological and Obstetrics consultant; Drs Doris Quinet, Gough, Israelski,

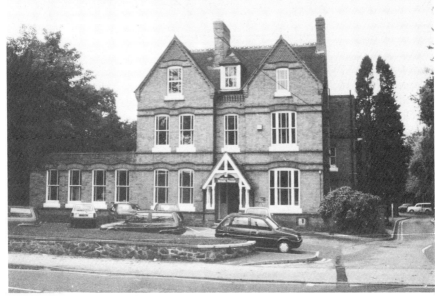

Brook House for many years part of the Maternity Department and now offices.   (JW)

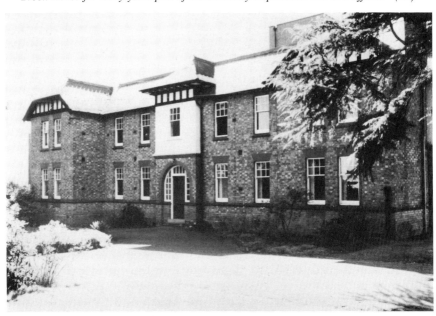

Catherine de Barnes Hospital built in 1910 for patients with infectious diseases. Later used as a Maternity home and finally for smallpox patients.   (SH)

Mary Crosse (Paediatrician), Jean Hallum (Gynaecologist), Thompson (Pathologist), Gillam and Nussey (Physicians) plus six resident junior doctors who were House Officers. Mr J. W. Riddoch and Mr J. S. M. Connell, surgeons who had previously worked at Eastcote Grange, also joined the team as did many others over the years. They were supported by professional and technical staff in the Dispensary, X-ray and Physiotherapy Departments each having two qualified full-time and one or two part-time staff. There was a visiting Chiropodist, Miss McGauley, who treated the in-patients, and a part-time Occupational Therapist — Miss Lewis — who did excellent work, especially with the chronic sick. Approximately 120 beds were available, more for women then for men, admissions running at about 330 per month. Miss Windridge, the Matron, and her assistant, Miss Tongue, had 65 full-time and 77 part-time nursing staff including 32 male orderlies. There were 12 administrative staff as well as the catering, cleaning and maintenance staff, altogether approximately 300 people.

'First class work . . . terrible conditions'

The Health Service was still in its infancy but already there were waiting lists although every effort was made to keep them down. At Solihull in May 1952, 221 people were waiting for operations plus 1,093 children who needed their tonsils removing. A major handicap was the condition of the wards; they were so dilapidated that washing the walls and cleaning was inadequate, even decorating was not enough for in places the wall plaster needed repairing. The wards were still heated by large stoves which blackened the ceilings and were difficult to sweep. There were no overhead bed lights, inefficient blinds and few wash basins, the nearest place for nurses on Ward A2 to wash their hands being three wards away. But the lavatories were worse, all being very old: in that adjoining Ward B2 the cistern splashed over and the pull damaged the plaster; that adjoining B4 had chipped tiles which had lost their glaze and the waste pipes of battered lead were much in need of attention. This was also the place where non-resident staff hung their coats. A lack of finance meant that only a little could be done at a time but by 1954 most of the wards had been painted and had new blinds fitted. New beds, mattresses, bedside lockers and bedpans were purchased and the chairs used for the up-patients were reupholstered or renewed. The other things had to wait until a ward's turn came for modernisation and repair. Despite all the problems the Hospital managed during 1952 to admit 4,650 patients, and undertake 1,068 major and 3,551 minor operations and open a special ward to deal wholly with the children's tonsils. As a member of a visiting party commented 'the hospital is doing first class work in terrible conditions which cannot improve without capital outlay. The same standards are demanded here as in places with better facilities'. The majority of patients were grateful for the treatment and care they received and many wrote to the Hospital with their thanks, some sending donations and one giving six dressing gowns to Ward B2.

In addition to the gifts donated by grateful patients, various groups in Solihull occasionally offered useful items. One of the earliest recorded came from the ladies of the Inner Wheel who in 1951 gave four chairs to Ward 3. This was followed by a portable altar for the Mortuary Chapel presented by the rector, Rev A. E. Fraser, the embroidered altar linen being given by the WVS. There was clearly a great deal of support for the Hospital in the town and an appreciation of the staff and their work. This resulted, in January 1953, in the formation of the 'Friends of Solihull Hospital' which the first chairman, Alderman W. E. Wright started off with a gift of £100. The Hospital management welcomed their interest and in April offered a place on the House Committee. The same year the Hospital purchased a tea trolley for the use of the Red Cross and this grew into a trolley shop which, manned by a rota of volunteers, took a variety of items to patients' bedsides. In 1954 the Friends began raising funds for specific projects, their earliest gifts being four garden seats, a piano and stool and a statue of Florence Nightingale. Thus began a long association which still continues and has brought many lasting benefits to the Hospital.

The Nursing Staff

There was some concern in July 1951 about the health of the nursing staff. Of the resident nurses, about half had been treated in the Hospital during the previous year, some for serious ailments. It was thought that many did not take care of their health, or eat enough, especially when on night duty, for they had to cook their own supper in the ward kitchens, if they had time; frequently they ate only a snack. Staff facilities generally were poor, there was not even an adequate cloakroom in the Main Block. A small first floor ward was used but it lacked secure lockers, sufficient coat hooks, or any privacy when changing. The night nurses used it as a rest room but it contained only a small gas fire and a couple of wooden chairs. There was a need, frequently reiterated by Miss Windridge, for a new Nurses Home with comfortable accommodation for 50 nurses. Their current home, Wayside in Lode Lane, was poorly heated and furnished with dilapidated chairs and a few carpets although improvements were being made. Eastcote Grange had been suggested as suitable for a Nurses Home, but it was too far from Solihull and lacking frequent public transport to be practical. Meanwhile The Beeches was being renovated and refurbished, at a cost of £2,700, for the use of the Matron and other nurses. The house was comparatively small but the work proceeded slowly and after three years was not wholly completed.

Miss Windridge was keen to start a Nurses Training School for she could foresee a serious shortage of fully trained nurses. Already Solihull had empty beds available but insufficient nurses, and at times orderlies were undertaking nursing for which they were not trained. Her plans for a school had been approved provisionally by the General Nursing Council (GNC) in 1950 but the BSOHMC needed to provide adequate rooms for lectures, demonstrations and study, as well as a Sister Tutor's office. In 1954 the GNC threatened to withdraw its approval if firm plans were not implemented within six months. Matron appealed to the BSOHMC and suggested that the Workhouse Guardians Board Room in the oldest part of the Hospital might be converted. She had already found three ward sisters who were capable of teaching the students. It took some time but in the end her persistence succeeded and the School opened on 1st January 1957.

Eastcote Grange and The Riddings

Some patients on leaving hospital went for a period of convalescence at Eastcote Grange. The house had been turned down not only as a Nurses Home but also as a suitable residence for the permanent inmates who although they lived at Solihull Hospital were supported financially by the Warwickshire County Council (WCC). The latter, however, refused to take on Eastcote and it was proposed that acute and chronic patients be sent there instead, but public transport was

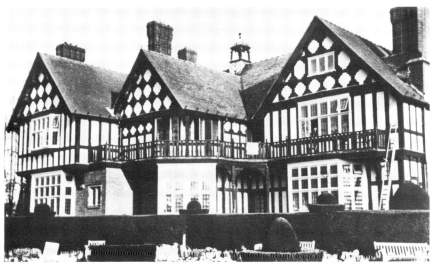

Eastcote Grange, known officially as the Midland Hospital.
After its closure it was sold and divided into luxury homes. (JRP)

again the problem. Finally the best use for the building, which had 34-36 beds and nursing staff accommodation, proved to be as a recovery hospital where patients could stay for two to three weeks. This relieved the pressure on acute beds at Solihull and sent patients home almost fully recovered. Opened in May 1952 and known officially as the Midland Hospital, between 40 and 50 patients

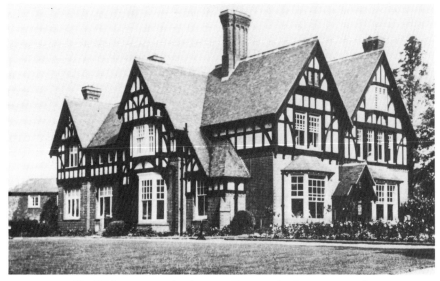

The Riddings, companion house to Eastcote, in the same grounds.
Similarly divided into homes.   (JRP)

per month were admitted. On fine days they could stroll and sit in the extensive gardens, gradually being restored after 15 years of neglect by one part-time and seven full-time gardeners. They planted shrubs and roses, laid paths with 10 tons of broken paving, and made a kitchen garden. Garden seats and deck chairs were purchased, the money coming from a special fund.

Parts of Eastcote needed refurbishing especially the kitchens which wanted new cookers and the worn and dangerous floor covering replaced. The patients' toilets and bathrooms also required improvement. Some of the staff lived in The Mews, a converted unheated garage dark and depressing in winter and damp. It needed power points, heaters, extra windows and the blue-brick bedroom floors covered with lino; it is a wonder any staff stayed. However, everything, apart from the heaters was deferred until The Riddings, another large house within the Eastcote grounds, was renovated to provide additional beds. The work took 18 months to complete, the first 11 patients being admitted in March 1954.

It was difficult to keep non-resident staff because of the transport problem. A cycle shed had been requested as some staff had bikes but it is doubtful if any, at this date, had a car. Solihull Hospital owned a vehicle which was used to ferry essential goods and people between Solihull and Eastcote but a close check was kept on its use; 9,763 miles being recorded in the 12 months to February 1954.

The Maternity Department

The Maternity Department at Solihull was divided between Brook House, Netherwood and Catherine de Barnes. The majority of births took place at Netherwood, the mothers and their babies being transferred within a day or two to Catherine de Barnes, this conveyor belt system working fairly well. It had come into being initially by force of circumstance, but it proved to be very safe and formed a new concept in maternity management. At Netherwood there were 16 beds, the staff coping with numerous stairs and a lack of wash basins, the patients accepting the crumbling plaster and dilapidated bedside tables without complaint. At Catherine de Barnes there were 28 beds increased to 36 in November 1953 by making efficient use of every space. Patients stayed about 12 days but by 1953 were no longer totally confined to bed. This necessitated changes in the bathing arrangements and it was suggested that the two baths in the main ward block might be supplemented by adding two shower attachments. Housing the staff was a problem and the idea that some nurses might lodge in private houses nearby was considered. During 1954 there was a shortage of technical, medical and nursing staff and the usual 18 midwives for both Netherwood and Catherine de Barnes was reduced to 15, causing admissions to be cut. On the whole conditions at Catherine de Barnes were quite good; there was central heating although in really cold weather it was inadequate and coal fires had to be lit in the wards making extra work. One of the kitchens also acted as sister's office where the telephone and patients' records were kept; this was neither hygienic nor private but a request for it to be partitioned was refused. However an application for a new sink and draining board, the existing one being in poor condition — which usually meant the porcelain lacked glaze and the drainer was decrepit — was considered.

At Brook House there was the usual lack of wash basins and a need for more and better sterilizing equipment. There were 17 beds available most being used by GP's, some of whom booked beds for their patients then failed to attend the birth. It was therefore decided to limit the number using the House to those willing to attend and who lived fairly near, a committee being set up to work out the details. A crisis occurred in April 1953 when a case of pemphigus, a potentially fatal skin disease characterized by watery blisters on the body, was found on a new baby. The baby and its mother were transferred to Little Bromwich Hospital for Infectious Diseases as were the further few cases which occurred. Admissions and visiting were stopped; where possible, patients were sent home and finally Brook House was closed and stoved, the staff being kept away from the rest of the Hospital and patients. All staff and patients were investigated including the porters and laundry workers. No source was found; but the swift and decisive action taken prevented further cases occurring: all the affected babies did well.

Following this serious infection it seemed sensible to decorate and renovate Brook House before reopening it; in all £4,500 was spent, the BSOHMC paying for the work. The back stairs were removed permitting some rearrangement of the rooms but the bulk of the work consisted of improving the sterilizing facilities, adding numerous basins with elbow taps, replacing baths and flattening dust catching moulded surfaces. The work took 14 months to complete even so not all that was planned and required was done. Brook House reopened in June 1954 when nine beds were ready. It was a time of midwife shortage, only 12 beds being open at Catherine de Barnes.

Altogether there were 63 Obstetric and Gynaecological beds in the main Hospital and the three Maternity Homes and the ideal for efficient nursing was a total of 26 midwives. Serious consideration was being given to the Hospital's ability to cope as the population increased and if the number of births rose as expected; a completely new unit was the only answer. In 1952, 897 babies were born to families living within Solihull UDC, the population of which was 68,420 and expected to rise to 100,000 by 1962. The Hospital also served Acocks Green, Sheldon, Hall Green, Barston, Hampton in Arden, Lapworth, Wythall and Earlswood which pushed the figures much higher; at least 70 beds were necessary, 20 for GP's and 50 for specialist obstetricians with a compliment of delivery theatres.

The Outpatients Departments

Many people visited the main Hospital in Lode Lane only as outpatients to attend clinics, the X-ray and Physiotherapy Departments and Casualty; the total number of attendances increasing from 48,000 in 1952 to 72,000 in 1953. The facilities, as elsewhere in the Hospital, were very poor, the staff in every department working in difficult circumstances and the patients suffering draughty primitive waiting rooms with inadequate toilets and little privacy. In the Chest Clinic two undressing cubicles were needed, one for each sex, but they were refused as being too costly; eventually they were allowed but by the time they were built the clinic had grown to 2,000 patients per annum. There were no washing facilities or a place where throat swabs could be taken. Finally a 12ft extension was built with two washbasins, three cubicles, lavatory and staff cloakroom. Physiotherapy managed very well but the patients' waiting room was a space under some stairs which was between two doors and very draughty. It was suggested it might be boarded in to make it more comfortable. The X-ray Department also had poor cubicle and waiting space which they somehow managed to improve. For a time in 1952 film was in short supply considerably reducing the department's work. When supplies improved the work rapidly increased and four full-time Radiographers were needed, although not always available. By the end of 1954 10,000 X-ray examinations were made per year and the department was on the priority list for an extension.

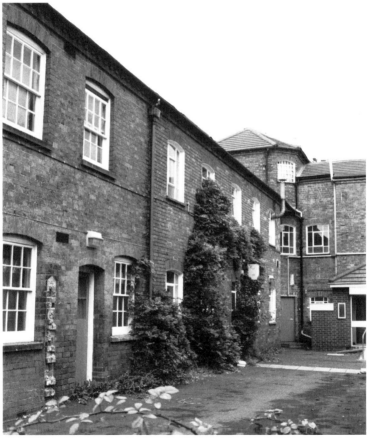

The tower and a wing of the oldest part of the Workhouse
used for many years by Pharmacy and the Pathology Department. (JW)

The Outpatients Department which then included Casualty and the Ante-natal clinics was under severe pressure with a cheerless cramped waiting room. An ingenious plan for increasing the number of undressing cubicles by incorporating part of the cycle shed was suggested, as was the erection of pre-fabricated buildings but the basic problem was financing any scheme. Early in 1953 a new Outpatients was on the future capital programme list, a year later it was upgraded to the priority list and might be considered in 1955/56. An accident in Lode Lane emphasised the paucity of facilities in Casualty, and yet despite the needs of a fast growing population it was 1959 before the new Outpatients department was ready.

It was usual at Solihull at this time for the nurses to take blood samples for testing. This was really a Pathology Laboratory technician's job but the Hospital had neither technicians nor laboratory. Until the latter could be established it was arranged that a technician, Mr W. A. Jones, should be ferried daily, Monday to Friday, by taxi to and from Selly Oak Hospital with the specimens he had taken. In the meantime a blood bank, containing cross-matched blood, was set up at Solihull and a small fridge purchased in which to store it. The work was important and increased as the number of patients and medical techniques grew, but not until 1954 was the Pathology Laboratory ready. Situated on the upper floor and in the tower of the Workhouse building it was opened by the Mayor-elect, Councillor R. D. Cooper. In the Dispensary, situated a floor below, the work also increased and more staff were needed, but suitably qualified people were in short supply. Space was a major problem, every inch of the Department being in use and saline solutions, penicillin and sulphur powder, which could have been made up quite cheaply, if there had been room in the laboratory, were bought in. A new Dispensary was put on the priority list for the financial year 1955/56 but with no idea when the work would be done. The rise in the number of operations and of medicines prescribed in Outpatients increased the Dispensary costs considerably. There were complaints about overspending but as more varied treatments and antibiotics became available it was only natural that doctors wished to use them. Fortunately economic expediency prevailed and having been enlarged and upgraded at a cost of £4,750 the Dispensary, from this time known as the Pharmacy, was opened by the Mayor, Councillor H. Moren-Brown in 1957.

Counting the Cost

Keeping down costs was a recurring theme; when in March 1953 the Hospital was found to be £10,500 over budget — the total running cost for the year being £161,000 — an investigation was set in hand. Every item of expenditure was examined in great detail. The cause proved to be nurses' salaries up £1,000, patients' food up £3,000, drugs, dressings and appliances up £2,000, fuel, light and laundry up £500, maintenance up £2,200 and repairs and renewals up £1,800.

The rises were the result of extra staff being employed to nurse more patients, a 10% rise in food prices and a better diet being given, as required by the Ministry of Health. The Hospital had no central heating but vast quantities of coal were used to heat the water and keep the many stoves going. It was estimated that (excluding the Midland Hospital) it cost £20.9.9 per week to keep a patient at Solihull, a rise of just under £3 in the year. Of this £15.15.9 was a standing charge i.e. what it cost to run and staff the Hospital whether there were any patients or not, and £4.14.0 was each patient's maintenance charge i.e. food, drugs, laundry, cleaning, use of linen, beds, utensils. Of the latter, food was the largest item costing £2.3.2 per week, well beyond the £1.4.0 stipulated by the BSOHMC. The Midland Hospital was also subjected to scrutiny, the total expenditure for 1952/53 being £21,500, £5,000 less than estimated. The staff, fuel, light, laundry and drugs bills were well under budget, the cost per patient being £15.8.8 per week. Convalescent patients needed few drugs but, as they regained their strength and appetite, a wholesome diet was recommended and £1.4.0 was insufficient to provide it. Similarly at Catherine de Barnes the new mothers required a nourishing diet with plenty of milk, but this cost £1.7.6. per week. The BSOHMC reiterated that £1.4.0 must not be exceeded and comparative costings with other hospitals in the group were put in hand. Except for the Accident Hospital, Solihull's costs were the highest, but unlike the others, it was a wholly general hospital and the comparisons were considered not altogether fair.

Stratford Hospital was then costed as being similar to Solihull, the towns being much the same size and with the same type of population. Stratford's costs proved to be less, at £16.6.4 per patient per week, but an average patient stayed 30 days as against 15 at Solihull. Acute patients cost the most to keep and nurse in the early stages of their time in hospital and transferring some cases to Eastcote to convalesce enabled Solihull to fully utilise every bed which almost certainly contributed to increased costs. It was also discovered that Solihull dealt with twice as many outpatients per annum as Stratford. However those holding the purse strings were still convinced economies could be made and suggested cutting the quantity of milk and greengrocery purchased. Undoubtedly everyone tried hard and only indented for the most essential equipment, such as a new washing machine (£550), when the parts for the old one were unobtainable. It had been purchased in 1928 and worked more or less continually for 26 years. Equally a new operating table (£510) was needed, the old one was to go to Casualty and the one there thrown out as obsolete and in poor condition. To pay for it the purchase of a cardiograph machine was deferred.

Patients and Staff

Thoughts were turned in November 1952 to celebrating the forthcoming Coronation without incurring great expense. Eventually it was decided to hire three televisions, two to be set up in the Dining Hall at the Hospital and one for Catherine de Barnes. The Council planned to decorate Lode Lane as far as Netherwood so £10 was earmarked for decorating the Hospital. During Coronation week a concert party visited the wards and gave a concert for those not in bed. On 1st June a special lunch of cold chicken and ham, fruit and ice cream with beer or cider was provided and the patients' visitors invited to tea. On the day itself Councillor Lines provided fresh eggs for breakfast, lunch was a cold buffet, followed by high tea, the decorated cake being provided by the Rotary Club.

For many years the Mortuary Porter and Post-mortem Assistant was Peter Stevens, a long-time resident in the Hospital having come there as a permanent inmate. Born about 1889 he had worked for several years in these posts, probably for little but his board and lodging. When the Health Service started in 1948 he was discharged as an inmate and taken on to the staff. By 1954 the Post-Mortem work was too heavy for him but he continued his Mortuary duties. A case of an outcast of society being found worthwhile work in a caring environment.

As the Hospital grew and the staff increased the permanent inmates were squeezed out of eating in the Dining Hall, now the canteen. Instead they had their meals in the sitting room of their own quarters but this was not thought to be either satisfactory or a proper way for them to be treated; consequently they reverted to taking meals in the Dining Hall. Instead it was the staff who moved to part of Ward E2 where hot beverages were available. This grew into a sort of staff canteen but it was not wholly suitable. It took several years to get a proper canteen but with the help of the Friends, who as their first big project raised £1,100, a wooden building was erected and fitted out at a cost of £4,500. It was opened in 1957, the old canteen reverting to a ward.

During the 1950's visiting times were subject to much scrutiny. In 1952 it varied throughout the Hospital and particularly in the maternity units where visits were limited to lessen infection. Brook House permitted husbands only to visit 7-8p.m. each evening and others on Wednesday and Sunday 3-4p.m. Netherwood and Catherine de Barnes allowed one hour visits two or three evenings a week and on Sunday afternoon. Poor public transport made the latter difficult to reach and many husbands had to walk home after visiting. In the rest of the Hospital short and frequent visits were thought best and in 1954 fixed at Wednesday and Sunday 2.15-3.30p.m., other days 7.15-7.45p.m.

The old public right of way from Lode Lane, which skirted the edge of the Hospital grounds, had been used for some years as the entrance drive. Patients were admitted through the Main Block and at night their arrival made considerable noise. It was suggested that new arrivals might be admitted at the rear of the Block through a door near the Operating Theatre. This led to the idea of an entrance from Union Road, for one-way ambulance traffic, if the Council would agree. In January 1953 a trial was begun, ambulances entering the grounds from Union Road through the old Tramps gateway and leaving via Lode Lane. It worked well and continued in use for many years.

Lode Lane at this time was narrow with high hedges and many trees, although there were gaslamps it was poorly lit. The Hospital drive was very dark with one light outside the Nurses Home but nothing more, and many of the female staff were nervous. The Council was approached and readily agreed to light it. So few people had cars that until 1954 there was no problem with parking but as their numbers increased it became more difficult, especially as most of the grounds were laid out in lawns and flower borders. It became necessary to remove the turf from an area near Outpatients and tarmac it.

Ten years on from the start of the Health Service much had been achieved at Solihull although much remained to be done. When, in 1957, The Mayor asked for the town to have a completely new hospital Alderman Bradbeer, Chairman of BSOHMC, spoke proudly of the £24,000 spent on the Hospital since 1948 and of future projects. Many thought the sum totally insufficient whilst others again expressed their appreciation of the work of the staff, despite the old buildings and poor facilities. The decade ended with a promise of a new Outpatients and improved Casualty Department, a remodelled laundry, modernised wards and a bed lift so that patients would no longer have to be carried manually up and down stairs.

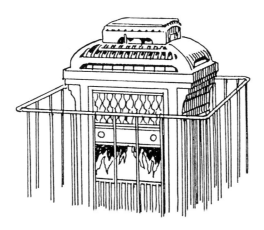

Drawing by George Busby of the type of stove which heated the wards until about 1965.

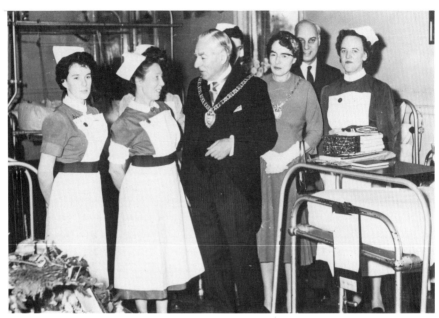

*Nurse Freeman chatting to the Mayor, Alderman H. Miller,
at the opening of Ward E4. Previously used as the canteen it was refurbished
to accommodate chronically sick elderly men.   (CJ)*

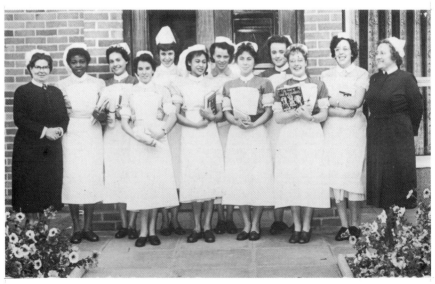

Prize winning nurses from the Training School, September 1959.   (SH)

'TOMORROW WILL BE BETTER'

The 1960's began on a strong note of optimism. The new Outpatients had opened recently as had Ward E4 and work was to begin shortly on reconstructing the Main Block and adding a bed lift and sun lounge given by the Friends. For the future there was hope of a new maternity unit, of new operating theatres and increasing the number of beds from 193 to perhaps 250.

The Outpatients, opened by the Mayor, Alderman H. Miller, faced onto Union Road and was situated partly in the Workhouse and partly in a new brick extension added to the front of the old building. Space had been made for it by demolishing a wing of the Workhouse which had proved to be unsafe. The greatly improved facilities made the staff's work much easier and provided seating for 40 in a bright and airy waiting room with a manned tea-bar in one corner; the total cost was about £30,000. The old Outpatients became the Casualty Department.

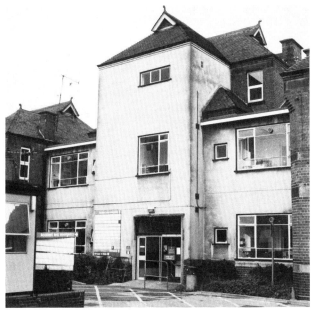

The entrance to the Hospital was altered considerably in the early 1960's to accommodate the bed lift. The plain rendering of this period contrasts sharply with the fine brickwork of the older part of the building. (JW)

In May 1960 the Friends gave the £3,000 they had raised to pay for the bed lift to the BSOHMC. This made it possible for work on the Main Block to begin almost a year sooner than expected, for only £1,000 had been allocated for capital work at Solihull during the 1960/61 financial year. The work was much more expensive than at first expected. It was completed and the Block re-opened in September 1962 the total cost, including the lift and sun lounge in the elderly women's Ward E4, being £34,000.

Solihull's status had changed considerably since the 1950's having become a Borough in 1954 and a County Borough in 1964 when the population reached 101,000; by 1966 it was 104,000 and still rising. Many of the newcomers were young and the three maternity units were under constant pressure. In 1960 the Hospital had more maternity bed bookings than it could cope with and many mothers-to-be were asked to have their babies at home if possible. The length of stay of those admitted was slightly reduced from the usual 7-17 days but the 'ruthless new practice of sending mothers home after 48 hours' recently started in Manchester and acclaimed by doctors there as 'sound medicine' was not introduced at Solihull. Instead the maternity staff struggled on under the guiding hand of Sister S. A. Richards who retired in 1964 and her successor Sister I. Michelson. When periodically the Hospital was threatened with closure it was this baby boom and the record of the Maternity Department which led to its staying open. Since the late 50's Solihull had qualified as a recognized obstetric training unit for doctors, and from the 60's a succession of medical students trained in the department, spending a month with Mr Hunt and Mr Watson helping with the delivery of babies.

A new Hospital Management Committee, Birmingham (Little Bromwich and Yardley Green) later known as Birmingham (East) was set up in 1962 and Solihull placed under its control. It had big plans for the future which included, as part of the Hospital Expansion Programme, the rebuilding and extending of Solihull Hospital so that 'in about 15 years most of the hospital would be completely new'. Because of the town's rapid growth, work would start in 1972 or before. In 1963 improvements costing £1 million were promised within five years: work was to start on a new maternity unit in 1966 and on twin operating theatres in 1967. By early 1964 plans for the former had reached an advanced stage and it was hoped that work on the unit, and indeed on upgrading the whole Hospital, might be brought forward. But nothing happened, and it was April 1966 when work on the £50,000 project began. Although it was not the complete Maternity Department dreamed of since 1954, the prefabricated post-natal recovery unit was extremely welcome and a step in the right direction.

Despite its problems Solihull had moved to the fore in a new and important service: screening for cervical cancer. Largely initiated by Mr Watson the work had begun in 1959 and by 1963 some 3,000 smears a year were carried out in the Gynaecological Outpatients Department. The service was extended to local area clinics in 1965, two technicians working under Dr R. H. B. Protheroe, the consultant pathologist, in the Hospital laboratory which was then dealing with 1,500 smears per quarter.

Another success was the resuscitation of Brother Bernard of Olton Friary. Feeling very ill in January 1966 he went to the Casualty Department where coronary thrombosis was diagnosed. Shortly afterwards he collapsed and his pulse ceased. Fortunately the Hospital had a new and expensive machine, a Cardiorater, which was used on him and his heart restarted. Few hospitals had such machines and Solihull had only one, but the dramatic story brought a swift response. The Rotarians immediately offered to donate a heart monitor and other groups joined in fund raising for additional Cardioraters.

Although the major building schemes were the ones which hit the headlines small but important improvements were going on continually. Ward 9, a prefabricated building, was erected in February 1964 and opened for female medical cases and in September two sun lounges were provided for Wards 6 and 7 by the Friends. In 1965 the female permanent inmates moved from the quarters they had occupied for so many years which were then demolished to make way for the new maternity unit. During the summer the Main Block central heating was extended and later the chimneys taken down and the Block reroofed. In December, Apsley, also previously used by the permanent inmates, was closed in preparation for conversion to a Nurses' Home. In 1966 the telephone trolley service, which had started in 1964 and enabled patients to telephone from their beds, was extended to Wards 3 and 4 and in time to all wards. Improvements and extensions were also made to the X-ray Department (£12,000) and a linking corridor donated by the Friends was incorporated.

Even so there were complaints: Solihull patients were obliged to travel to the Eye Hospital in Birmingham or to Selly Oak for eye treatment as Solihull had no clinic. Some GP's considered this too difficult especially for old people with cataracts or glaucoma and too far for children. Those with squints had to attend regularly and this was disruptive of their school day. Although the nursing was highly praised, the food in the maternity units was criticized by some new mums. They thought it unimaginative and too stodgy for those confined to bed all day, the quoted menus including veal and ham pie, fish cakes, and spaghetti, all served with mashed potatoes. Some grumbles were understandable; it was a shock for those male surgical patients who, in March 1965, were admitted to a warm, bright modern Ward 3 to find themselves transferred, post-op, to a cold, drab Ward 4 with its peeling paint, ill-fitting windows which the snow penetrated and ancient decrepit toilets. Mr R. J. Bugg, the Hospital Secretary, agreed that the ward was sub-standard but explained that large waiting lists made its use a necessity. Shortly afterwards central heating was installed and the ward

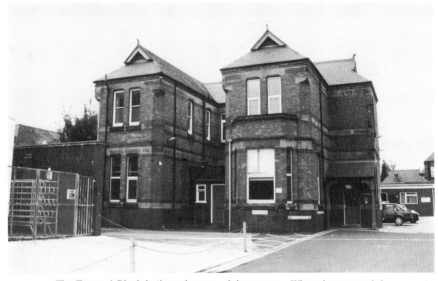

The Tramps' Block built at the turn of the century. When the tramps left, the ground floor became Outpatients and later Casualty. (JW)

decorated. The following winter there were serious complaints about Casualty which was often virtually closed in the evening and at weekends, and for a time could only deal with fractures on a Friday. For several years the Department was at a very low point, staff was difficult to get and keep, the post of Casualty Officer not being regarded highly. The facilities left much to be desired being described by one doctor as 'like an adapted stable' and there is little doubt that public confidence was badly dented.

In the spring of 1966 there was an outbreak of smallpox in the Midlands and it was decided to return Catherine de Barnes to its original use as an isolation hospital. Within 48 hours the maternity patients and staff had been moved out, walls knocked down and new beds and equipment, including mobile incinerators and disinfection materials, moved in. Two miles of barbed wire were run round the perimeter, four strands high and 'Keep Out' signs erected. All patients in the Midlands were transferred there and it became the Regional Smallpox Reserve Hospital. The first two Solihull patients were admitted in July.

During the early 60's four people who had given many years of service to the Hospital from its earliest days retired. Doris Quinet in 1960, Mr Wilson, the Hospital Secretary, in 1961, Miss Windridge in 1965 and Mr Quinet officially the same year but he continued to work in the Hospital for some time afterwards and was greatly touched to have Ward 1 named after him. Mr Wilson was succeeded by Mr Bugg and Miss Windridge by Miss Margaret Dicks.

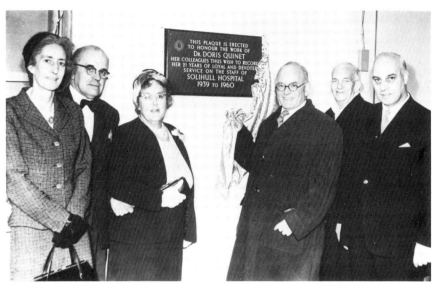

Dr Doris Quinet, centre right, at the unveiling of a plaque in her honour.
She is accompanied, left to right, by Miss J. Hallum; Mr Paul Quinet;
Dr Featherstone, senior anaesthetist at the General Hospital;
Alderman Bradbeer, chairman of BSOHMC and Mr H. Watson.   (HBW)

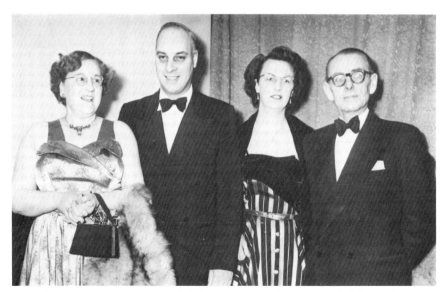

A pleasant evening at a Hospital Ball in the early 1960's enjoyed, left to right,
by Miss Windridge, the matron; Mr Harold and Mrs Barbara Watson and
Mr Horace Wilson, the Hospital Secretary.   (HBW)

51

Promises, Promises...

In May 1966 revised Government plans for midland hospitals were announced: Solihull was to be completely rebuilt at a cost of £1 million, offering first class maternity and general care in 700 beds; work would start in 1967 and last several years. Little Bromwich Hospital, increasingly known as East Birmingham, was also to be extended considerably, to become a District General Hospital with 1,200 beds; the cost would be £3 million. Already it dealt with 13,000 patients per annum, sharing consultants with Solihull. Until both hospitals were completed there was little hope of reducing waiting lists.

Since Solihull had come under the aegis of Birmingham (East) Hospital Management Committee (BEHMC) considerable improvements had been made including £40,000 spent on X-Ray equipment but from this time progress seemed to slow down. The following years were ones of national financial difficulty but East Birmingham Hospital and others saw many of their plans completed in full. Whilst at Solihull the attainment of the new hospital seemed to slip further and further away although the land for it was available, having been purchased with great foresight by the Local Authority in 1961. But as 1966 closed three projects were scheduled to start shortly; a Casualty Department, a Nurses' Home and the long awaited Maternity Block where the whole Department would be under one roof. It was to have 100 beds and form Phase 1 of the new hospital.

Early in the new year the Nurses Training School celebrated its 10th birthday and Mrs Davies, the principal Nurse Tutor since its foundation, retired. She had taught 93 nurse pupils, all but one passing the two-year nursing course. There was still a shortage of trained nurses but it was hoped the new Nurses' Home would help recruitment. In July 1967 the first turf of the site was cut by student nurse Joyce Martin who shared a room in the existing Home. The new building, expected to cost £53,750, was to house 24 nurses in single bed-sitting rooms. When it was completed, the old Home would be demolished to make way for the Maternity Block.

Nurses spent about three hours each mid-day serving food to patients from bulk containers and clearing away. A newly introduced system relieved them of this task. Patients chose their lunch from a menu submitted at breakfast time. Placed on a heated trolley the meals were distributed by waitresses. At Brook House the meals, cooked in the Hospital kitchen, were wheeled across the road by porters. Unfortunately they sometimes had to wait five minutes for a break in the traffic.

Since 1965, because of the shortage of midwives, all births had taken place at Netherwood, patients then being transferred to Brook House or, since Catherine de Barnes closed, Marston Green Maternity Hospital where Solihull had the use of 20 beds. Three quarters of births in the Borough in 1965/66 took place in a maternity unit where stays were, of necessity, now only five or six days. Consequently the opening of Ward 10, the prefabricated 20 bed post-natal recovery unit, on 8th March 1967 was particularly welcome. The first mother and baby were Mrs Brenda Abbey and her son Howard, transferred from Netherwood. Pleasant and comfortable with pastel walls and matching lockers the unit was carefully planned — a trial run for the projected Maternity Block — it had a stainless steel 'baby bar' where nursery feeds were dispensed automatically into hygienic disposable bottles, plus many other innovations. Patients were asked their opinion of the unit and encouraged to suggest improvements.

During 1967 and 1968 there were occasional press reports about the new Hospital (Phase II) which, it was believed, would be started soon. It was expected to include a 60 bed psychiatric unit, children's wards, operating theatres, extensive laboratory space and an intensive care cardiac unit. In the meantime, in October 1967, an extension to Outpatients was opened, £5,000 having been spent improving the chest clinic and on providing a psychiatric clinic, thus saving some patients the long journey to Hollymoor Hospital at Northfield which treated Solihull's psychiatric cases. Unfortunately, work on the desperately needed Casualty Unit, then scheduled to begin, was deferred for the design to be enlarged.

The new Nurses' Home opened in June 1968; it had central heating, two communal sitting rooms, a kitchen, and each bedroom had a washbasin and built-in wardrobe. The design was versatile, the rooms being easily convertible to two-room flats. Each room also had an electric fire and fitted carpet laid over a plastic tiled floor. To have both central heating and a fire, plastic tiles and carpet was regarded by some as extravagantly luxurious in frugal times, but this was refuted, for the whole project was completed for £45,000. The nurses themselves thought that they deserved to be warm and comfortable after so many years in sub-standard accommodation.

During the summer a complaint that a ten year old girl, a patient in an adult ward, was helping to 'nurse' post operative patients as they recovered consciousness, led to a spirited correspondence in the local paper on many subjects related to the Hospital. Chiefly these were the unsuitability of children in adult wards, visiting times — still the same as in the 1950's — and the shortage of nursing staff. Many ex-patients, once again, hotly defended the medical treatment and nursing, and the chairman of BEHMC said Solihull spent more on staff than other hospitals, but all agreed there were still many shortcomings such as the lack of a children's ward, and insufficient geriatric facilities. The disbanding of the House Committees, which included local lay people, was also considered a retrograde step.

The Beeches was relinquished to the Local Authority in September, and in

October a block of changing rooms containing two large locker-rooms and four cubicles was opened. A gift of the ever generous Friends (£3,500), they were intended for the use of the 70-80 non-resident nurses who had previously changed in odd rooms all over the Hospital. The next year the Friends provided bedcurtains for the five wards still without them (£1,500). Alderman Wright, now their President, had in December cut the first turf on the site of the Maternity Block which was scheduled to be completed in 1971. Shortly afterwards the old Nurses' Home was demolished, Netherwood having to be closed for 10 days because of the dust.

A Training School for Midwives was started in March 1969, the first floor at Netherwood being refurbished to provide two classrooms, a clinical room and an office for the Midwife Tutor. There was room for 10 students on the six-month course which was intended to provide qualified staff for the new maternity unit.

A very special birthday was celebrated in September when Mrs Eliza Moseley, who had been a patient since 1958, was 103. A party for fellow patients in Ward 8 was attended by Miss Dicks, the Matron, and other staff. Sadly Mrs Moseley died two months later.

...Always Promises

Solihull had 364 people waiting for surgery in 1966. To help reduce the numbers, day surgery for minor cases had been suggested but many doctors had mixed feelings about patients going home so quickly after an operation.

From 1968 the waiting list had grown steadily to reach 950 by February 1970, operations having been cancelled at short notice throughout 1969 due to a shortage of beds. Even so 5,589 people were admitted to the 216 beds and there were 54,000 attendances at Outpatients and Casualty during the year. At this time it cost, on average, £45.1.5 per week to keep a patient in Solihull as against the national average of £43.11.1.

Solihull was not the only hospital with a huge list; throughout the Birmingham area, demand was outstripping beds and facilities, a desperate shortage of funds leading to major delays in the building programme. When Richard Crossman, Secretary of State for Health, said more money should be given to the Midlands and North there was anticipation that building might be speeded up. Detailed plans for several projects, including Operating Theatres, intensive care, Pathology and X-ray Departments, kitchen and staff quarters, were already drawn up and during 1970 work on a number began; the long deferred Casualty Unit in June and a kitchen development in November. Ward 4 was upgraded in July and an intensive care unit started in Ward 1 in August. A new Boiler House, costing £115,000 with a 120ft concrete chimney, was ready for use in October, but it was the only one of the above structures which was to be permanent, the others were all temporary, the best available until the original plans could be implemented.

The increase in building and the growing number of cars made parking difficult and doctors and ambulances frequently could not get through. Eventually a car park was made off Union Road on rough ground beyond the Boiler House.

After being delayed twice through lack of equipment, the Casualty and Accident Unit finally opened in January 1971. Adjoining Ward 5 it had cost £25,000 but as a morale booster for both staff and patients it was worth much more. The bright, airy surroundings, large reception area with telephone and cloakroom, up-to-date equipment and resuscitation bays were in sharp contrast to the dark, cramped conditions which prevailed in the old unit. Piped oxygen and gas, instead of cylinders were now available as were trolleys on which patients could remain whilst being X-rayed or treated. Unfortunately by the summer the unit was on the verge of closing at night and weekends for lack of Casualty Officers and was only kept going by junior doctors doing overtime and by G.P.'s, the latter having played a vital part during the staffing crises of the last few years. There was a general shortage of doctors prepared to undertake casualty work; the reasons were many, but low pay, long hours and low professional status played a major part. There were still insufficient nurses, and cleaning staff were becoming scarce as they were tempted into domestic work by housewives who offered 10s per hour, much more than the Hospital could afford.

During 1971 a gastroscope and monitoring system (£2,000), used to detect the early stages of stomach cancer, were given to the Hospital by the Friends. A temporary Operating Theatre, installed in a tent, was opened in June whilst a more permanent theatre was being built. Large enough to carry the full range of equipment and five staff, the tented Theatre, similar to those used by the Army, had plastic walls and its own sterilisation unit and air-filtration system. Placed in the disused Casualty Unit it cost £13,000 and was expected to be in use for a year. A temporary corridor, bridging the yard, joined the tented Theatre to the Main Block. Work on the permanent theatre, adjoining the existing one, had begun in May but as the work progressed the medical staff were disturbed to learn that it would not have a piped supply of medical gases but cylinders which were cheaper. They were also concerned about the inadequacies of the Pathology Laboratory and suspected that following the recent improvements and the completion of the Maternity Block, which was imminent, development would cease for many years, especially when they heard that £2½ million was to be spent at East Birmingham. Solihull was once again the poor relation. Mr Percy Grieve, Solihull's MP, took up the matter with the Minister and the Birmingham

Regional Hospital Board (BRHB); assurances were given that Phase II would go ahead, but no date could yet be given.

Rosalind Stevens, née Shelley, the rhesus baby who made medical history in 1945 when her blood was changed, came to Solihull in 1971 to have her own baby, Katherine, under the supervision of Mr Watson. At the end of the year Sister Marion Pinckney retired, aged 68, having been a nurse for 50 years, always in midwifery, and for the last 10 years at Netherwood. At the same time the contractors, W. J. Whittall and Son Ltd, completed the Maternity Block, which after fitting out, would open in the spring.

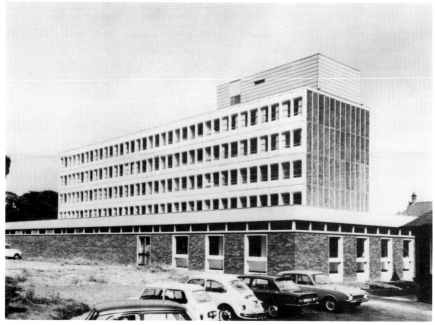

The Maternity Block shortly after its completion in 1972. (SH)

The opening of the Maternity Block was the great event of 1972, indeed one of the most important since the Hospital started, for this new expensive but vital unit — the first multi-storey permanent building for patients since 1910 — ultimately ensured the future survival of the Hospital. Of reinforced concrete and five storeys high it contained 112 beds in four wards, one on each of the upper floors. On the ground floor was a central delivery suite, full of the latest equipment for the use of consultants, GP's and midwives, the Operating Theatre and adjoining recovery ward, a premature baby unit with 14 cots, suites of consulting and examination rooms, a laboratory and the Outpatients Department.

Also on the ground floor was the Midwifery Training School and in the huge basement the new telephone exchange for the whole Hospital. The Midwifery School had moved in early in the new year when 120 nurses and a full complement of ancillary and secretarial staff were recruited. Then at 8a.m. on 10th April 32 mothers-to-be were transferred to the Block, the first baby, Alex Komoroczy, arriving at 11.10a.m., the event being later marked by the gift to him of an engraved silver spoon. As soon as the new occupants were installed Netherwood, Brook House and Ward 10 were closed. The latter was refurbished and opened in the following September as a general surgery ward.

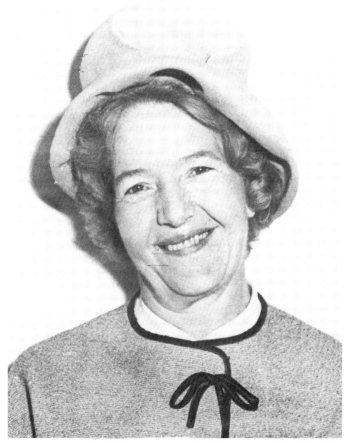

Sister Hilda Wood who ran the Casualty unit at the Hospital.
She retired in October 1972 after working at Solihull for 23 years.   (HBW)

A subject of much discussion at this time was the use of the pain killing epidural block during childbirth. It had been available at Solihull since 1966 but only in general use since 1970. Administered by an anaesthetist who has received special training, the epidural method numbs the lower half of the body whilst the mother remains fully alert. As its use increased there were complaints that it was sometimes given unnecessarily and a few mothers felt deprived, emotionally. Miss J. Hallum, the consultant gynaecologist, joined the debate, her view being that childbirth was becoming altogether too scientific. However, by the early 1970's epidural block was an established procedure which greatly improved the safety of both mother and child. It revolutionised the delivery of breech babies and Caesarian births, with the result that fewer babies needed resuscitation.

In the spring of 1972 Staff Nurse Carol Taylor became Personality Nurse in the finals of the Heart of England Nurse contest organized by the British Heart Foundation. By answering general knowledge and medical questions and projecting a pleasing personality Mrs Taylor won £150, a holiday and heart equipment worth £500 for Solihull Hospital. With the money a heartbeat trend recorder was purchased and presented to Carol, for use in the proposed Coronary Care Unit (CCU), by Des O'Connor who had spent some days in such a unit a few years previously. With the help of the Friends and other groups who were launching appeals, the Hospital hoped to set up a mixed four bed CCU, the number of heart deaths in Solihull being particularly high (53.6%), but each bed cost £1,000 plus, approximately £12,000 being needed in all. The BEHMC was willing to give £3,000 but the rest had to be raised.

In September the new Operating Theatre suite was completed and in October the Duchess of Gloucester was due to visit Solihull and officially open the Maternity Block. Sadly her elder son, Prince William, was killed in a flying accident and the opening was deferred.

Meanwhile a starting date for Phase II was still awaited. Mr Grieve, despite all his efforts, had failed to get a definite answer but the implication was that nothing would happen before 1976; he could get no promise of anything earlier. The medical staff were severely disappointed; they were also worried about the kind of service they could offer the public if there were further delays in the building programme. The Pathology Laboratory was an area of particular concern; patients who attended grumbled and thought it a disgrace, but felt most sorry for the staff who worked in such ancient and cramped conditions. A new laboratory was promised in Phase II but as such a long wait was now expected it was decided that short-term improvements costing £12,000 would be made; in the event only £1,000 was spent.

The Government announced changes in the running of the Health Service to take effect from 1974 when local goverment would also be reorganized. The

Regional Hospital Boards would disappear and be replaced by regional health authorities and, at local level, area health authorities which would work alongside the new local councils. Despite assurances there were fears at Solihull that this shake-up might set back even further the start of Phase II. There were to be changes too in the care of the mentally ill who were no longer to be treated and housed in large institutions but in general hospitals and the community.

During the summer there were complaints from ladies passing the Hospital that smuts from the Boiler House chimney had fallen on them and their nylon tights had disintegrated. The boiler and chimney were inspected but the evidence was inconclusive and the probable cause was thought to be the boiler being turned low during the summer.

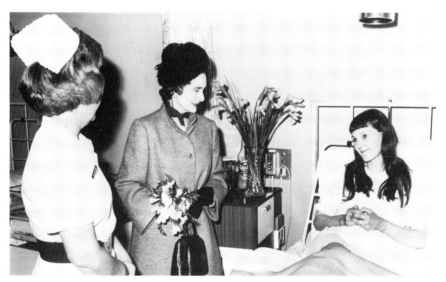

The Duchess of Gloucester chatting with a patient and Sister Winifred Knight at the official opening of the Maternity Block on 10th January 1973. (Courtesy Birmingham Post and Mail)

The deferred opening of the Maternity Block by the Duchess of Gloucester took place on 10th January 1973. Following an inaugural lunch for 250 at the St. John's Hotel the Duchess drove to the Hospital and made a thorough tour of the new building, chatting to the mothers and staff and admiring the babies. She watched the feeding of some premature babies in the special care unit before going on to inspect the Midwifery Training School. A commemorative plaque in the foyer was unveiled by the Duchess who said she was greatly impressed by the unit and its excellent amenities, a 'truly magnificent addition to Solihull Hospital'. Already it was proving to be a huge success, 1500 babies having been born there since it opened.

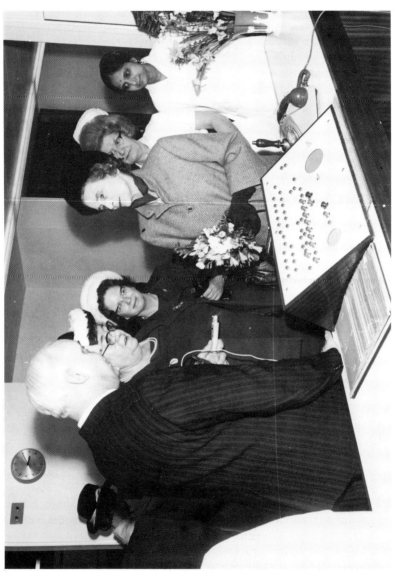

Mr Watson explains a technical point to the Duchess when showing her round the Maternity Block.
Also present, left to right, Miss M. Maxwell, principal nursing officer; Dr M. Barton, consultant paediatrician;
Sister Knight and another member of staff.   (Courtesy Birmingham Post and Mail)

DARKEST BEFORE THE DAWN

The Difficult '70's

The completion, fitting out and opening of the Maternity Block had given all concerned a sense of satisfaction and achievement but it was set against a background of national industrial unrest. There had been power cuts in December 1970, a postal strike in 1971 and, just before Christmas 1972, a one day strike by hospital ancillary workers over a wage agreement, in which the Solihull workers joined. Two months later in February 1973 industrial action was again threatened by the hospital workers and this developed into lightening and then full strikes, which stopped all but emergency services for a month. Solihull did not suffer as badly as many hospitals, the full strike lasting only a week during which some laundry, operating theatre and switch board services were maintained, but waiting lists were badly effected and grew even longer. There were threats of more strikes, and at Solihull a serious shortage of nurses which, it was feared, might result in wards being closed. To combat this a 'nurse bank' was begun; the scheme was designed to encourage qualified nurses with families to return to work, their hours being flexible to fit in with their domestic commitments.

During the year several groups and organizations raised money for equipment for the Coronary Care Unit (CCU) although work on it had not yet begun. By July, when the contract was finally placed, the costs had escalated so much that the BEHMC share had risen from £3,000 to £14,500. Work began in the autumn, the unit, attached to Ward 7, opening, at last, in March 1974.

It was feared that Government spending cuts would defer even longer the start of Phase II. Assurances were given that this was not so, but dissatisfaction with the lack of progress was voiced throughout the Borough. When, in July 1973, talks between the Department of Health and the BRHB confirmed that there was no chance of Phase II starting before 1976 and, furthermore, was 28th on a list of 34 projects planned up to 1981/82, it became real anger. Local organizations suggested that a petition with 50,000 signatures might bring about a change of mind, but nothing, apparently, could do that.

Almost the only good things about 1973 were the opening of a day centre for psychiatric patients situated in the refurbished old police station at Hobs Moat and, in December, the opening of three new residential blocks for medical staff, erected in Grove Road at a cost of £93,000.

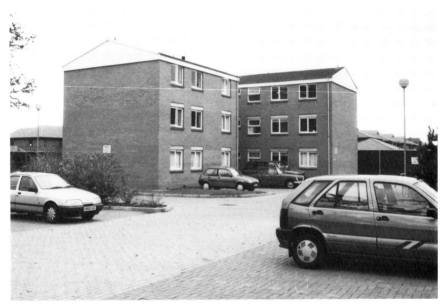

One of the medical staff residential blocks built in Grove Road. (JW)

In April 1974 Solihull became a Metropolitan Borough (SMB), the area under its control doubling in size and having a population of 200,000. At the same time Solihull Area Health Authority (SAHA) came into being. The same size as SMB it had four chief officers but no office, no staff or equipment until space was taken in Radcliffe House and Clarendon House, both recently built office blocks. The SAHA, working alongside the Local Authority, was to be responsible for a new system of community care and, through various committees and management teams, for clinics, practices, health centres and hospitals.

At the Hospital, with Phase II still far in the future, more make do and mend measures were put in hand. A Casualty Theatre was added to the Accident Unit in December 1974, Ward 1 was converted to Orthopaedic and Trauma in March

1975 and the Dickensian Pathology Department was upgraded in two phases both being completed by November 1975. Space as ever was difficult to find and from December the medical secretaries were housed in a Portakabin.

Matt Munro, the popular singer, broke his collar bone in a fall when appearing in a Solihull nightclub in January 1976. He was taken to the Hospital where he was treated, signing his X-rays for the radiographer, Janet Musgrove.

The ongoing national economic problems which included high inflation and difficult labour relations, meant cuts, go-slows and strikes occurred from time to time throughout these and subsequent years, money always being in short supply. At a meeting held in Birmingham in May 1976 a bleak picture of the Health Service in the West Midlands was drawn by doctors and consultants — declining standards, crumbling buildings, insufficient staff. About the same time the SAHA reorganized the Solihull Hospital 'nurse bank' system, cutting their permitted working hours. A consultant surgeon, Mr Robert Holl-Allen, deplored the move as these nurses played a vital part in keeping the Hospital going and he refused to do major operations if enough qualified nurses were not available on the wards to care for his post operative patients. Matters were smoothed over temporarily but other consultants agreed with him and were generally dissatisfied with the way the Hospital was funded. They were critical of the size of the administration and felt too little money was going into patient care. The controversy was increased when Miss Susan Atkinson, the principal Pharmacist, complained of the appalling conditions in which she and her staff worked. Still housed in the oldest part of the Workhouse the Pharmacy had walls which held dust and prevented the making of certain sterile fluids, other fluids were stored in a lean-to shed, whilst volatile stores were kept in an old air raid shelter. The lack of a cool room meant some drugs could deteriorate. There was little hope with the present funding, of the Department moving to better accommodation for many years — perhaps as long as eight.

At an enquiry into the running of the SAHA, it emerged that the Authority was in considerable financial difficulties, its £8½ million budget being £160,000 overspent in 1974/75, £428,000 in 1975/76, the estimated deficit for 1976/77 being £268,000. The rent for the offices in Radcliffe House, which the Regional Health Authority (RHA) had advised against taking as too expensive, was £105,000 per annum. In addition £4,588 had been paid to consultants for office layout and £30,000 spent on setting up the offices. The rent for the two floors of offices in Clarendon House was some £30,000 per annum, one floor being left empty. A huge row broke out between the various bodies involved which rumbled on for well over a year. The SAHA was advised to leave Radcliffe House and move to Brook House which had recently been renovated, but the Local Authority would not allow this as it was in a residential area, although at a later date they relented. The Council offered two floors of offices in the old Council House in Poplar Road at a reasonable rent which would save £75,000 per annum, and a house, 83 Homer Road, was also taken. To save money, short term, all-round cuts of 5% were ordered which the Hospital found difficult to manage — patient and staff meals were effected, which caused some concern, whilst a cut in the porters' overtime slowed down the working of the whole Hospital and had to be restored. The closing of various centres was suggested, the largest saving being made — £50,000-£100,000 per annum — if the Midland Hospital was included. This caused a terrific outcry as the recovery unit at Eastcote increased the number of patients treated at Lode Lane and a stay in rural calm helped many patients to recover more quickly. But in spite of the protests the Midland was closed, temporarily, in September 1976. From this time, patients who needed to convalesce were sent to Marston Green but they were not so happy there as it did not have the lovely garden or the atmosphere of Eastcote. The staff, who felt they had been somewhat curtly dismissed with no farewells or thanks after years of service, hoped the Hospital would open again, but it never did. After being mothballed for two years it was officially closed in 1978. By pruning all round, including the number of pupil midwives in training, the projected deficit for 1976/77 became a saving of £96,000. It took two enquiries into the SAHA to sort everything out; by the end one chief officer had taken another post, three were suspended or soon left and the chairman was replaced. The other Authority members were dismissed by the RHA, against government orders.

This unpleasant episode excited considerable discussion amongst doctors, councillors and the public about the Hospital. For the present it could only deal with the needs of a quarter of the 200,000 population in general medicine and surgery and only 15% in geriatric requirements. For dentistry, paediatrics, ear nose and throat (ENT), ophthalmology and mental illness, it was necessary to go elsewhere. There were insufficient beds, the back-up services continued to struggle in ancient buildings and the Pharmacy closely resembled a slum. Apart from the Maternity Department hardly anything had changed in 18 years. Some GP's thought that with the large, modern and well-equipped East Birmingham Hospital so close, it was unrealistic to expect Solihull to offer an equal service, but the majority of the residents supported Solihull whole heartedly, including Mr John Black, the new chairman of the SAHA, who was determined the Hospital would improve and grow. In July 1977, at a crowded public meeting in the town, the Friends launched a fighting fund of £200,000 under the banner — Campaign for Action on Solihull Hospital (CASH) — and decided to send a letter of protest to the Department of Health and the RHA demanding immediate improvements at the Hospital. During the autumn the RHA, answering questions put by the Residents Association and reminded of numerous previously broken promises, said work on improving the Hospital would start in 1983 and by 1985/86 there would be a new building on the Hospital site. This reply, if not wholly believed, was encouraging but when, a few months later, the RHA put out its 'Strategy for Health' Solihull was not even mentioned, and ignoring SAHA's plans to start building in 1983, had shelved Phase II for 10 years.

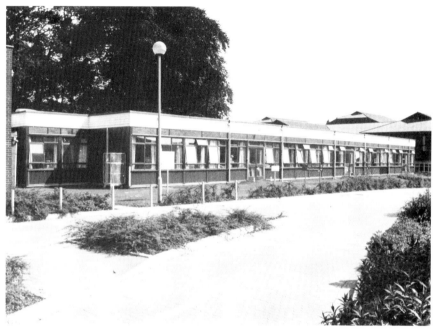

Apsley, the unit for the elderly, opened in October 1977.   (JW)

In 1975 Apsley was pulled down and a single storey unit, providing a range of services for the elderly, built in its place. The new unit, retaining the name Apsley, was bright and airy and contained 38 beds plus two day-rooms for in-patients. It also catered for 25 day-patients; physiotherapy, occupational and speech therapy, chiropody, dietary advice and rehabilitation assessment being available. The elderly men and women from Wards 6 and 8 moved to the new unit prior to it opening in October 1977. The original intention had been to insert a lift in the old building, up to Ward 6, on the first floor to which patients had always been carried. But to spend £70,000 on an outdated building when £180,000 would provide a comfortable, spacious, purpose-built unit seemed false economy. A year later Ward 6 was reopened as a staff changing room and in May 1980 Ward 8 as an acute medical ward, the cost of its refurbishment being £95,000.

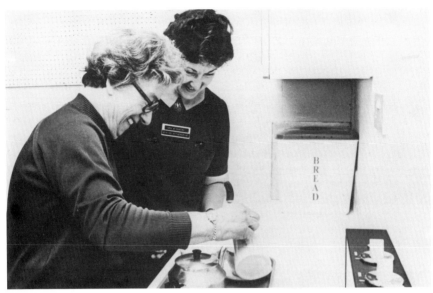

*Mrs Shirley Hanlon, the Head Occupational Therapist, and Mrs Ivy Allkins,
one of the first of the day-patients, enjoying a cup of tea in the kitchen
of Apsley shortly after the unit opened. (Courtesy Solihull News)*

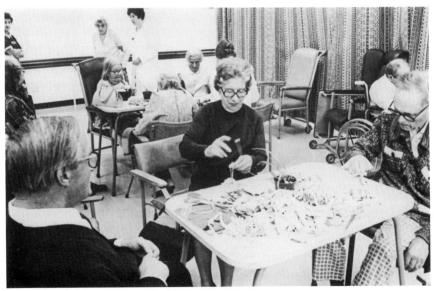

*Apsley patients, both day and residential, busy with their occupational therapy.
Mr John Newman, left, and Mrs Ivy Allkins, centre, the unit's first two day-patients.
(Courtesy Solihull News)*

Since 1976 and the debâcle of the SAHA overspending, various groups in Solihull had shown their support for the Hospital by raising money for special items of equipment. Mr A. J. Polyzoides, an orthopaedic consultant internationally acclaimed for pioneering a new operation on wrist joint replacement, was one of the early recipients, when the ladies of Knowle and Dorridge Inner Wheel presented him with £400 to buy vital joint replacement equipment. Subsequently many people were extremely generous and hard working raising large sums for sophisticated monitors and machinery, much of which was very expensive. The Friends continued to provide their much needed support giving, as always, their time and approximately £20,000 per year in funds.

In February 1978 Netherwood, where so many Silhillians had been born, was demolished to make way for a single storey Physiotherapy Department which was to be built adjoining the Maternity Block at a cost of £200,000. Containing a gymnasium and a vast array of up-to-date equipment the unit opened in December 1979. The wooden hut in which it had been housed for several years

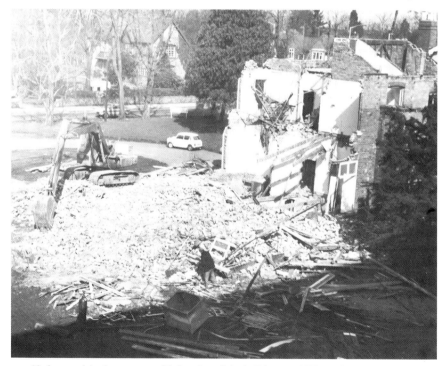

Netherwood in the process of being demolished, February 1978 Lode Lane is in the background and beyond is the house where Paul and Doris Quinet lived in their retirement. It was demolished in 1989 and the site is now covered with retirement flats.
(Courtesy Solihull News)

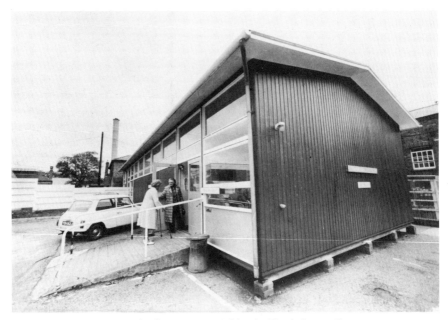

For many years this hut was occupied by the Physiotherapy Department.
Later part of it became the Chiropody Clinic. (SH)

was taken over by other departments including Chiropody, there being a huge demand for the treatment of foot problems and 300 people waiting for attention in 1978.

In August Mrs Janet Parker, a medical photographer working in the medical microbiology laboratory at Birmingham University, developed smallpox and together with several colleagues was sent to the Isolation Hospital at Catherine de Barnes. The others were cleared but Mrs Parker, who caught a particular virulent strain, died. She was the last known person in the world to die of the disease and in 1980 smallpox was declared officially eradicated. Even so the Hospital was kept in a state of readiness for several years, meticulously cared for by Mr and Mrs L. Harris, the caretakers.

Since the closure of the Midland Hospital the buildings and grounds had become something of a white elephant. As in the 1950's, the distance from Solihull and poor public transport limited their use. Many doctors would have liked the Hospital reopened and used once more for convalescent patients, but this was refused as being too expensive and selling the property was discussed. For a time it was used by the Save The Children Fund but finally, in the early 1980's, Eastcote and The Riddings were sold and divided into apartments to provide luxury homes.

The hopeful '80's

A Health Service reshuffle took place in April 1982, 22 new health districts being created. The idea behind the changes was to give greater control in the daily running of hospitals and the spending of resources to team managers, doctors and nurses. Solihull, within its existing boundaries, became a health district and with a budget of £20 million per annum was in future known as Solihull Health Authority (SHA).

Shortly after these changes took place there were again national threats of strikes and some industrial action over hospital employees' pay. Solihull was effected and for a time only emergency patients were admitted. The Hospital had huge waiting lists for orthopaedic surgery, particularly for hip joint replacements, the consultants at Solihull having a very high national reputation. Unfortunately the Orthopaedic team had only three sessions of operating theatre time per week and 24 beds for their patients. In order to try and reduce the list which then stood at 700, two further theatre sessions per week were transferred in June 1982 from Gynaecology to Orthopaedics. The latter also needed more beds but these could not be surrendered by Gynaecology for fear it would lose its recognition as a training department for junior doctors, a given number of beds being necessary for this recognition.

Mr Harold Watson retired in July 1982 after 41 years at Solihull. His staff and colleagues, past and present, gave him a farewell party to acknowledge his years of devotion to the Maternity Department and to the Hospital for which he had done so much.

Having considered the matter for four years, the RHA finally agreed early in 1983 that Solihull ought to have a fully viable hospital on its own doorstep and that it should not be a mere satellite of East Birmingham, as it was at present, but should be upgraded to a District General Hospital; Solihull being the only Health Authority in the West Midlands without a hospital of this status. To reach this standard it would need a further 135 acute beds, proper facilities for children and the elderly and huge improvements in most departments; indeed a complete overhaul or the long promised rebuild, if the Hospital was to serve the people properly. So much which had been renovated, renewed or built over the years was now becoming dilapidated, out of date or superseded by new medical techniques. The work was expected to cost £10 million and, if the DIISS would give its approval, start in 1987. The supporters of CASH were delighted and staff morale was greatly boosted.

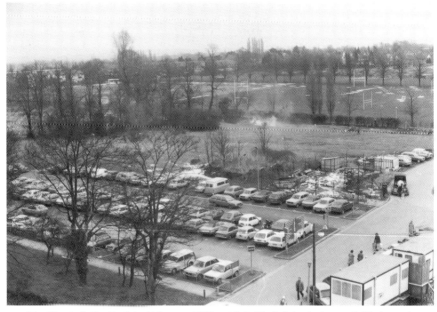

The Hospital Car Park in February 1983, with Solihull School playing fields beyond.
The new Hospital now covers the area.   (Courtesy Birmingham Post and Mail)

1983 was also a bumper year for appeals; several groups and clubs raised funds to buy machines and equipment, including a foetal monitor and neo-care incubator, for the ante-natal clinic, the Special Care Baby Unit and other departments. In September the largest appeal ever made on the Hospital's behalf, for a laser for the Gynaecological Department, was launched. It was to be used in the treatment of cancer of the cervix. The laser cost about £19,000 but the target was £35,000 in order to cover the running costs. The Mayor, Mrs Miriam Harris, launched the appeal and within a few weeks it had reached £4,000. The local press gave it generous coverage and collections, raffles, disco's, fun-runs, car-washes, darts matches and many other activities boosted the fund week by week. The target was reached, through the public's generosity and good will, in just over six months, half the time it was expected to take. Money continued to be raised, however, long after the target date and was most gratefully received.

Unfortunately 1983 was also a year of staff cuts. A women's surgical ward was closed and the waiting lists grew longer but the renewed hope of the new hospital cheered everyone.

The national shift from enrolled nurses to State Registered Nurses (SRN) led, in 1984, to a reduction in the number of nurse-pupils in the Training School. SRN's needed detailed training in specialities which Solihull could not provide

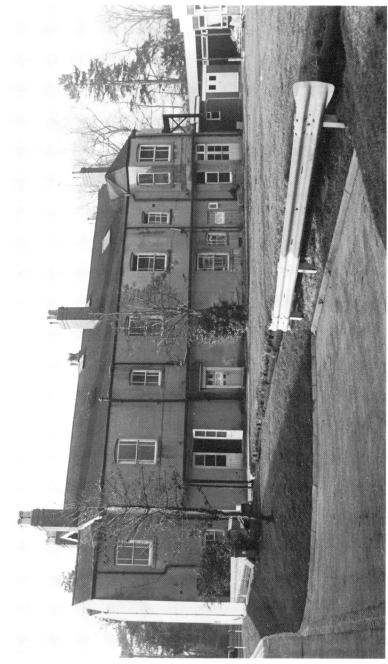

The rear of Ardenne demolished in 1984. The low building of the new Apsley can be seen at the right. (Courtesy Solihull News)

until the Hospital was extended and its services for both patients and staff training developed. During the year the nurses in the Accident and Emergency unit elected to change their uniform and, for practical reasons, wear trousers instead of skirts: navy for sisters, royal blue for staff nurses and bottle green for enrolled nurses.

Ardenne, the last of the row of houses in Lode Lane which had served the Hospital so well, was demolished in March 1984. The site was cleared in the expectation that the Hospital redevelopment would cover the area and the car park behind. The RHA, however, was talking of further delays which sparked

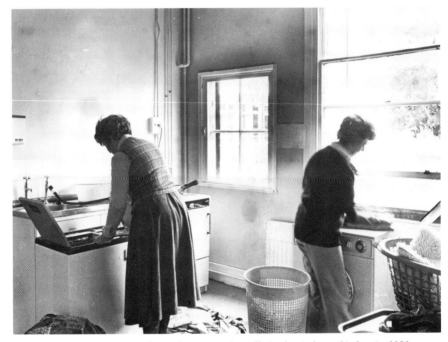

WRVS ladies washing the Apsley patients' smalls in the Ardenne kitchen in 1981.
(Courtesy Solihull News)

off a storm of protest throughout the Borough. In May and June the local newspapers were full of articles and letters setting out how desperately the District General Hospital (DGH) was needed. The cost had risen to £22 million but in July the RHA agreed to a September 1988 start, but there were warnings that the battle was not yet finally won, for annual reviews of its 10 year plan might lead to further delays. Within a year, a start in 1991 was being discussed; there were renewed protests, a petition and the Borough's two MP's — John Taylor for Solihull and Ian Mills for Meriden — went to see John Patten, the junior Minister of Health, who gave them a sympathetic hearing and agreed to put their

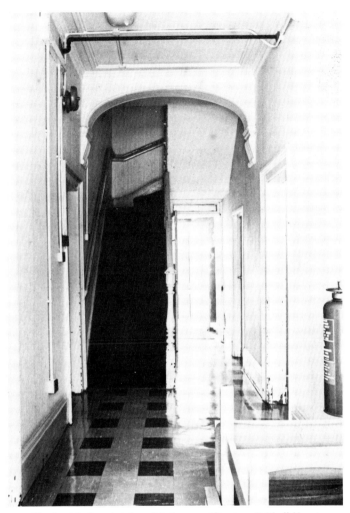

The front hall and stairs of Ardenne. *(Courtesy Solihull News)*

objections to Mr James Ackers, chairman of the RHA, but 1991 it remained.

At the end of 1985 Catherine de Barnes Hospital finally closed. It had been kept empty, but ready to take smallpox patients at four hours notice, for seven years, even though the disease was officially eradicated. The site was sold soon afterwards and the buildings converted into private residences.

During the year a number of improvements took place at Lode Lane including the refurbishment of Ward 9 which reopened in September and the completion of an ultrasound computer for the Maternity unit, a gift of the Friends.

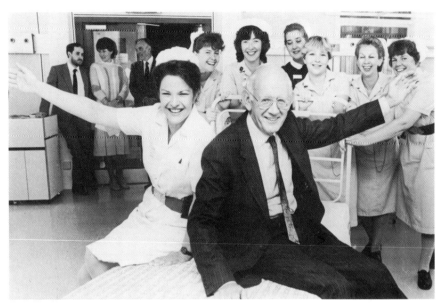

Ward 9, newly refurbished, was reopened in September 1985. Here nurse Manager Sister Turner and Mr John Black, chairman of the SHA, are given a lift by, left to right, Staff Nurses A. Thompson and Sarah Perrins, Sister Julia White, Enrolled Nurse Anna Capes, Auxiliary Nurse Janet Bayliss and Staff Nurse Thelma Hepple whilst Graham White and Dr Robert Montgomery discuss more serious matters with an unknown lady.
(Courtesy Solihull News)

' . . . but the end is not yet. '

The promise of the DGH, even if its realisation was some way off, together with the success of the appeals which demonstrated tremendous public support for the Hospital, produced, from about 1985, a subtle new sense of purpose. Positive improvements in anticipation of the DGH resulted. A spacious new Pharmacy, at least 20 years overdue, opened in January 1987 and two months later a new Outpatients, also greatly needed, came into use. By the autumn however, partly due to inflation and pay awards, financial constraints were necessary, the SHA being considerably overspent. A number of cost cutting options were considered and those chosen — the closure of the 17-bed convalescent unit at Marston Green, and also the Accident and Emergency unit at Lode Lane at night — were highly criticized. Both decisions were much regretted but particularly the latter which meant that from 30th November all those in Solihull needing emergency treatment between 8.00p.m. and 7.30a.m. had to go elsewhere, to Birmingham, Warwick, Redditch or Coventry.

The Orthopaedic Department's extra operating sessions had been a help but not enough to reduce the waiting list which was now one of the longest in the country. Something had to be done especially to improve the bed provision. Consequently, in January 1988, aided by an £150,000 donation from the Government and a considerable degree of co-operation between the medical staff, a 24-bed orthopaedic ward was opened. Two consultants and additional nurses were engaged for the ward, where it was hoped an extra 500 patients a year could be treated. By 1990 the Department had eight operating sessions and five Outpatient clinics a week, the waiting list had been considerably reduced and 71% more in-patients treated. As a result it was decided to undertake hip and knee joint replacement operations for a number of patients from Shropshire. The decision was criticized by some, but the Department earned £20,000 with which physiotherapy sessions could be improved and an extra set of orthopaedic instruments purchased. Shortly afterwards a party of 10 Brazilian surgeons came to Solihull specially to watch Mr Polyzoides demonstrate the 'rotor glide total knee replacement' operation and fit an artificial joint, the design of which he

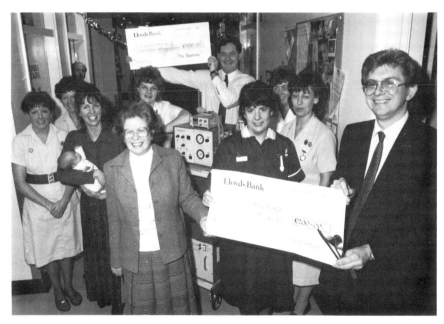

Dr Margaret Barton receives a cheque in December 1988 for £200 to pay for a meal for the 32 staff of the SCBU, a Christmas present from grateful parents. A larger cheque for £1,200 was also presented by Steve and Ian Burton whose nephew, Thomas, weighed only 1lb 14oz at birth and was cared for by the unit. Ian, at the rear, holds the cheque aloft surrounded by parents and staff. (Courtesy Birmingham Post and Mail)

had developed eight years previously, to a patient. Following the hour long operation patients spend three days in bed before undergoing physiotherapy; on the fourth day they can walk and after 12 days are able to go home.

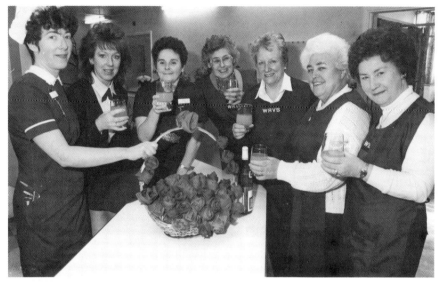

In February 1989 Ward Sister Katie Tapson gave a party for her 'part-time angels', ladies of the WRVS who helped her with non-medical tasks on Ward 10. Here, left to right, Sister Sarah Perrins, Mrs Lynne Lee, Sister Tapson, Mrs Olga Legg, Mrs Hazel Ferrari, Mrs Gladys Stansbie and Mrs Vickie Rayner raise their glasses. (Courtesy Birmingham Post and Mail)

The wonderful response to the Laser Appeal which ultimately raised £75,000, more than twice the target amount, was followed by other fund raising efforts by the public: an electro-cardiograph machine for the Accident and Emergency unit, and a £3,700 life support machine, both to replace ones that were almost worn out. A generous gesture by a former patient, Miss Carlotta Cohen, who left £125,000 to the Hospital, made it possible for a new clinic to open within the Physiotherapy Department early in 1988. Named after Miss Cohen, the clinic was able to treat 25 arthritis patients each week. Other gifts during the year included nebulizers to assist breathing, two accident trolleys, and several large sums to buy specialist equipment for the Special Care Baby Unit where premature babies, some weighing as little as two pounds, received care.

A further major appeal, for £100,000, was launched in November 1988 to set up a centre for women and families in four areas. To be known as Care 4 there would be clinics for infertility, cervical cancer laser surgery, baby assessment and menopausal problems. Some of these services were provided already but often the facilities were quite inadequate. The centre would be set up in an unused area of the Maternity Block and open in 1990. Here a much needed menopause clinic would be started and a separate cervical cancer clinic for which demand was growing. This would enable women whose smears showed abnormalities, a most stressful time for them, to be seen, and if necessary treated, in calm and relaxed surroundings rather than in the busy ante-natal clinic as at present. An infertility clinic would expand the existing service and give the benefit of new techniques to infertile couples, whilst the baby assessment unit would enable the Hospital to improve and expand its 'follow up' treatment of premature and low weight babies. About 300 of the 3,000 babies delivered at Solihull each year are tiny and admitted to the Special Care Baby Unit. Subsequently they need prolonged monitoring of their growth and development.

The Care 4 Suite opened to patients in January 1990, the official opening by Lady Jayne Ackers, the wife of the chairman of the RHA, taking place in April when the total sum raised stood at £120,000. Lady Ackers paid particular tribute to Dr Chris Stockdale, a Shirley GP, who raised £12,000 by a sponsored swim of 30 miles across Lake Garda in Italy.

The Hospital chimney was again causing trouble in October 1989 when its black smoke, the result of burning dressings, clinical, theatre and hospital waste, was noted by environmentalists. The whole of Solihull was shortly to become smokeless but as crown property the Hospital was exempt from the regulations, a matter of some concern to them.

Since the late 1980's there had been a positive effort to make the Hospital more patient friendly and less institutional. Ordinary furniture, and wall paper made the long stay wards more homely, the patients wearing their own clothes which were washed for them by the staff in a well equipped laundry. A flower stall opened near the Maternity unit, a hairdressing service was introduced and individual headphones for those wishing to watch TV without disturbing other patients. The Reception staff were trained to make attending hospital less daunting and doctors encouraged to discuss with their patients the plan for their care and the procedure for treatment. There was special concern and help for the bereaved, a quiet room and a trained welfare officer being available.

In 1988 the National Health Service was 40 years old and the following year, on the anniversary of the outbreak of the Second World War, the Hospital itself was 50 years old. In those early days few could have imagined the major developments which would take place in medicine, of the conquering of killer diseases — TB, pneumonia, diphtheria, smallpox etc. — and of the long and intricate operations which surgeons would be able to perform. Neither could they have guessed at the huge sums which would be spent on the nation's health. For the founders of the NHS firmly believed that, by offering free care to all, the people's health would improve so greatly that demand would fall away and within a few years the cost would diminish.

'...A LITTLE MORE PATIENCE...'

In the autumn of 1988 it was confirmed that the DGH would definitely go ahead and a few months later there were suggestions that its construction might start ahead of schedule. The plans and a model of the Hospital were unveiled to the press in January 1990 and soon afterwards put on public display. Work was due to begin in October but it was December before the first turf was cut. Baroness Hooper, Parliamentary Under-Secretary of State for Health, performed the ceremony using a JCB instead of the traditional spade, although a commemorative silver spade was presented to her. This she returned to John Clark, the Hospital General Manager, who pledged to put it on permanent display when the building was completed. In her speech Lady Hooper said that she was aware that the idea of the Hospital had 'been germinating for a very long time. All you need now is a little more patience to wait for the completion date in 1994.'

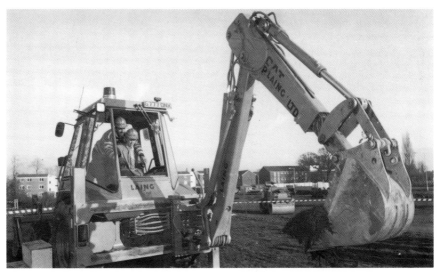

Baroness Hooper cutting the first turf of the DGH with a JCB,
assisted by the machine's driver. (Courtesy Birmingham Post and Mail)

In the many years since the Hospital was first envisaged much has changed in attitudes to health care, comfort and pleasant surroundings being well to the fore. The DGH, estimated to cost £34 million, will be decorated in pastel colours and have good quality carpets and furniture. The design makes the best use of natural light and the windows will look out onto several courtyard gardens. There will be 400 beds including 124 for the elderly, 81 for surgical patients, 60 for the mentally ill and 14 special care cots. Also planned are a new X-ray Department, Pathology unit, four new Operating Theatres, an Ophthalmology Department, Dental and Orthodontic units, a child development clinic and an Education Centre for nurses and post-graduate doctors. The latter will have a tiered lecture theatre seating 110, a library, and class and meeting rooms where medical and technical staff can meet regularly with consultants in their own speciality and in other fields.

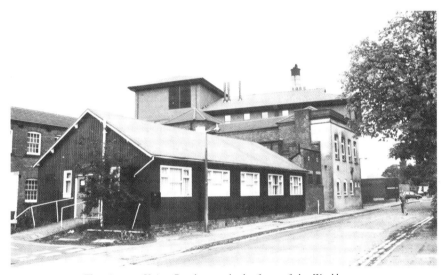

The view up Union Road towards the front of the Workhouse, rendered over in the 1960's. The wooden building was erected with the help of the Friends in 1957 for use as a canteen. The new Pathology Block towers over the old buildings.   (JW)

In the meantime the acute services were being expanded in readiness for the DGH, an ENT clinic had opened in February 1989 and a 20-bed maternity ward, which had been closed for some time, was reopened. In order to make the best use of the beds available a short stay surgical unit was opened in Ward 4 early in 1990. For both men and women it dealt with general surgery and urology cases, opening at 7.30a.m. each Monday and closing at 8p.m. each Friday, some patients staying for only a day.

Since cars had become more numerous, parking at the Hospital had been increasingly difficult. It became even worse when charges were introduced in the town centre parks and selfish workers and shoppers parked in the Hospital grounds rather than pay. The situation became very serious, delaying ambulances and doctors. Despite warnings and appeals the problem continued and in 1984 clamping was tried but not until 1990, when barriers were set up at a cost of £25,000 and a charge of 50p introduced, was the problem brought under control. The relatives of long stay patients and those on low incomes together with many outpatients complained bitterly about the charges, but the strategy worked and shoppers and office workers ceased to park in the Hospital spaces. For those in real need a system of free tokens was devised.

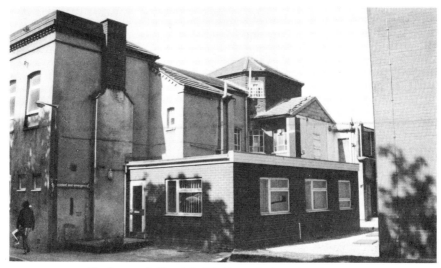

The front and side of the Workhouse looking the other way.
On the right is the edge of the new Pathology Block and centre,
the remains of the Workhouse wing pulled down to make way for it.   (JW)

There had been concern for some time about the high rate of deaths in the Midlands in babies under a month old, 6.8 per thousand dying in Solihull as against the national average of 4.9 per thousand. Poor ante-natal care was thought to be a possible factor with the prospective mothers not taking sufficient care of their health. Despite a detailed survey the exact cause was not pin-pointed but smoking and a poor diet appeared to play a major part, many pregnant women failing to give up or even cut down on smoking and alcohol. In order to provide better communication between mothers-to-be and the health care staff, Dr Ralph Settatree, consultant obstetrician at Solihull Maternity unit, pioneered a scheme to give women their own health records — notes on medical history, test results, scans etc and pages where they could jot down queries and their own notes — thus giving them a greater role in their pregnancy care.

Early in the year a suite of rooms away from the bustle of the Maternity Block was opened for the use of the parents of very sick babies. Comfortably furnished and decorated with funds raised by the maternity staff, it provided a quiet peaceful home from home.

In March the Special Care Baby Unit (SCBU) launched a competition inviting children to design a SCBU logo which could be used on mugs and T-shirts. These would then be sold at the Hospital to raise funds. Twenty children entered designs which were judged in May by consultant Dr Watkinson, local artist Alfred Steadman and one of the Friends; the winner was Rachel Smith, aged six.

A radio station, Solihull Central Sound, especially for the Hospital patients and staff, made its first broadcast in May 1990. Manned by young volunteers who raised £2,000 plus to buy equipment, the station has a studio and office at the Hospital. Started in a small way the volunteers plan, in the future, to operate a 24-hour service every day. They will relay messages from family and friends and visit patients on the wards to ask them what they would like to hear. The station is not intended to compete with the Birmingham Hospitals Broadcasting Network, but to supplement it.

In June 1990 there were suggestions that a crèche should be started at the Hospital to attract working mothers into nursing to ease staff shortages. Not enough school leavers were going into nursing, a profession which was already short staffed and which too few men were entering. One problem was the number of other attractive professions open to women. A direct entry midwifery course, eliminating the need for initial nurse training, was about to begin at the Birmingham and Solihull College of Midwifery Education, whilst at the Queen Elizabeth College in Edgbaston a number of student nurses were being trained especially to work at the DGH in 1994. It is hoped that the new Hospital with its increased technology and Education Centre will attract more trainees.

The expectation of war in the Gulf hung over January 1991 like a black cloud. Casualties were expected to be heavy and many would be flown to England for treatment. An appeal for extra blood donors was met by a huge public response and hospitals were asked to make preparations. Solihull set aside a ward where less serious or orthopaedic casualties might be treated. Fortunately casualties were light and the war was quickly brought to an end.

A major new appeal had been launched in 1990 by the *Solihull Times* under the title 'Pulse'. On behalf of the Hospital it was asking for several pieces of medical equipment, including a video system for use in endoscopic operations (£15,000), an Opmaster theatre table for the Accident and Emergency unit (£3,000), a Curapulse for use in Physiotherapy (£4,000), a mobile cardiac defibrillator (£4,300), a voice communication aid for stroke damaged patients

(£2,000) and an incubator for the SCBU (£4,000). The newspaper suggested that clubs and organizations might adopt one of the items on the list and raise the necessary funds. Almost immediately a generous widow, Mrs Eileen Dewar, gave the Opmaster table in memory of her husband, and numerous individuals and groups donated the monies from their annual fund raising events to the appeal. In addition generous people continued to make gifts to the SCBU. A pair of special scales by the Purcell family, money from Cubs, schools and pensioners plus £2,500 from a failed band who gave the proceeds from the sale of their instruments.

A special picnic for Teddy Bears, their owners and families was organized by the *Solihull Times* at the Norman Green Athletic Centre in August 1991, over £1,000 being raised in under three hours. Later, *Solihull Times* readers raised a further £600 and the total sum was used to buy a Photo Therapy Unit where premature babies with jaundice can be treated. The unit bathes the baby in special light which relieves the condition caused by the production of too much bile.

Mr Polyzoides was again in the news in 1991, his Rotaglide Total Knee attracting surgeons to Solihull from around the world. They attend the workshops which are given quite regularly at the Hospital to demonstrate the operation. The three piece knee unit copies nature precisely and allows the knee to rotate and twist reducing strain on the joint.

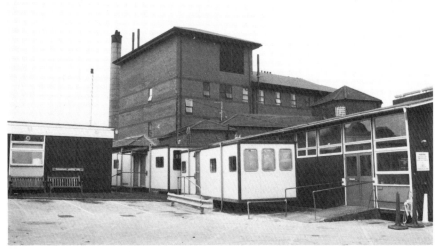

The hotch-potch of buildings, old, new and temporary
which, in 1993, serve the Hospital.   (JW)

After six months work the DGH was well under way and on schedule. The old main entrance drive from Lode Lane was shortly to be closed off and a new one, closer to Apsley, opened. The car parks would be improved with patient and visitor spaces close to the Hospital. A new staff car park had been made behind Brook House although many nurses leaving the Hospital after 10p.m. were very nervous about using it. The problem was finally resolved by permitting them to park nearer the Hospital. The new buildings rose very quickly and had reached the topping-out stage by July 1992 when Sir James Ackers visited Solihull to perform the ceremony.

Increasingly, patients were having their operations carried out on a day surgery basis, almost one in three being done in this way at Solihull. In May 1992 ENT treatment and surgery for children on a day basis was introduced. The aim was to do 30.5 operations of all types in this way per day but a 10% higher rate was achieved. Unfortunately the number of patients waiting for bladder surgery had increased considerably and operations were undertaken on a Saturday to try and reduce the list. This was a success and by also using available empty beds and operating time in other hospitals, the list had been cut considerably by May 1993.

The Drive for Excellence

The Solihull Hospital Foundation, a registered charity, was set up in April 1992 to establish 'a permanent Trust Fund for today's and tomorrow's requirements. Requirements beyond Health Service funding abilities.' The Foundation's aim is to make the DGH a model of medical achievement by providing considerable financial help from the community — companies and professional firms, charitable trusts, schools, sports and social clubs, families and individuals. In return the donors will have their names displayed in the relevant area, and the knowledge that they have made a worthwhile contribution toward what all hope will be a centre of excellence.

A generous response was received, Glaxo Laboratories giving £10,000 for an endoscope to be used in the gastroenterology unit, and the Heart Association a £7,000 Treadmill, which helps detect angina, to the Electrocardiogram unit. A Shirley based firm, H.V. Skan, gave £50,000 to provide an intensive therapy unit and the Central England Training and Enterprise Council donated £14,000 to the Education Centre, part of a £28,000 donation by an anonymous company.

The logistics of keeping the Hospital working whilst joining the old to the new were quite complex. The old Outpatients, including the wings of the Workhouse, had been demolished so that the new Pathology Laboratory could be built. Finally, in May 1993 after almost 40 years in its cramped quarters

THE NEW SOLIHULL HOSPITAL

Health Service funding in excess of £35 million

The Solihull Hospital will attract the finest professional staff giving top-class healthcare benefits to the local community.

Benefits which the people of Solihull EXPECT, DESERVE AND ARE DETERMINED TO ACHIEVE

BENEFITS THROUGH PARTNERSHIP

The Health Service with the people of Solihull can create

A CENTRE OF EXCELLENCE

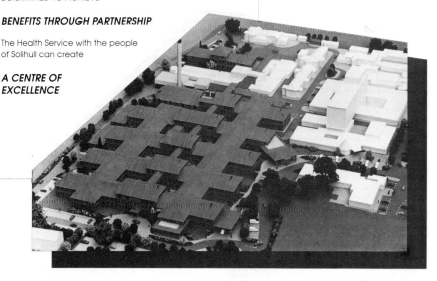

The Top Ten Priorities of equally vital equipment are listed below. With this equipment the Hospital staff will have the wherewithal to deal with the widest range of patient-care.

Choose your level of donation and associate your name with any of the following:

* Infertility Laser Scanners £30,000
* Infant Life Support Ventilators £25,000
* Children's Hearing Test Equipment £20,000
* Smear-Test Screening Microscopes £10,000
* Ante-Natal Screening Monitors £25,000
* Cardiac Resuscitators £25,000
* High-Speed X-Ray Cameras £20,000
* ECG Machines £10,000
* Cardiac Monitors £5,000
* Stroke-Patient Treatment Beds £5,000

Extracts from the Solihull Hospital Foundation brochure asking for financial support from the community. (SH)

NHS funds
need supplementing by
establishing a
PERMANENT TRUST FUND
for today's and tomorrow's
requirements.
Requirements beyond
Health Service
funding abilities

Requirements
YOU AND YOUR ORGANISATION
could be proud to provide

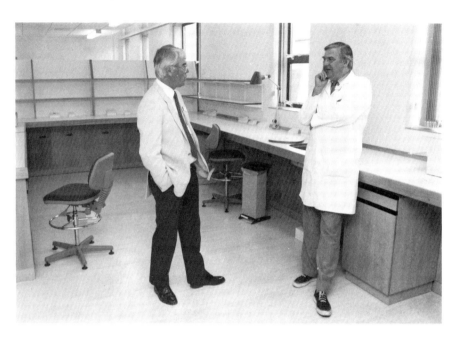

▲

The new Pathology Department shortly
before its opening in May 1993.
Jim Page, Head Medical Laboratory
Scientific Officer of the Haematology
Department,in discussion with
Mike Ellis, the Laboratory Business
Manager.
(Courtesy Birmingham Post and Mail)

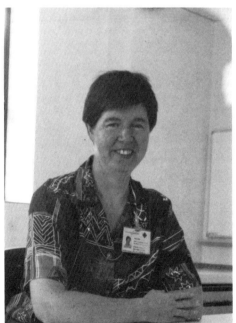

◀

Yvonne Langton, Medical Laboratory
Scientific Officer, Cytology Department,
in her new laboratory in the
Pathology building.
(Courtesy Birmingham Post and Mail)

in the old Workhouse, the Pathology Department moved to a purpose built three storey building next door. Although the staff of the various departments looked forward to working in modern clean premises not everyone was happy to see the old buildings go, Councillor George Benson being anxious to keep the Workhouse tower even if none of the other buildings could be retained.

A further appeal to sponsor a bed in the DGH under the Name a Bed Scheme was launched early in 1993, £1,000 paying for each one. Groups and societies who could raise such a sum were happy to respond and by November 60 beds had been sponsored, Laing Midlands, the builders of the DGH, being one of the first to give their support.

The Hospital is very keen to have a body scanner, essential for the rapid and painless diagnosis of certain types of cancer and brain disease. The cost, £500,000, is huge and requires a special kind of fund raising. In May, with the support of the *Solihull News* which gave generous publicity, the Scanner Appeal was launched. 'Skangaroo' badges — a kangaroo shaped lapel pin — are being sold for £1 each in shops, pubs, clubs etc throughout the Borough. Schools are also actively involved, £7,000 being raised within the first week. The appeal continues and it is very much hoped that the target will be reached by the time the DGH opens in 1994.

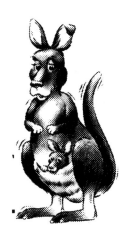

The people of Solihull have waited a long time for their Hospital. For decades they showed great patience and for the past few years enormous generosity and support for the staff and medical teams working in a hotch-potch of buildings which make up the present Hospital. But the new 'centre of excellence' is nearly ready and the dream is almost realized.

Sources and Bibliography

Doris Quinet, *Paul Quinet* (1982) pp 31-38

Solihull Parish Accounts St Alphege Church 1657-76, at Warwick County Record Office. Ref: DRB64/

Solihull Parish Church Warden Accounts 1724-8 at WRCO

W. E. Tate, *Parish Chest* (1960)

Solihull Workhouse Records at WRCO CR51/

Birmingham University Extra-Mural Group 1960-74; Unpublished papers

Craig D. Stephenson, 'Victoria's Bastille? a case study of a Warwickshire Workhouse, Solihull 1836-1901', *Warwickshire History,* vol vii No. 1 (1987)

Directories

Solihull Hospital Archive

Key to Caption Credits

Reproduced by kind permission of:

SB	Sue Bates
NF	Miss Nan Freeman
BG	Dr Brian Gough
DG	Dr Denis Gray
JRP	J. R. Pettman
HBW	H. B. Watson
JW	John Woodall
A	Aerofilms Ltd
Birmingham Post and Mail	The Birmingham Post and Mail Ltd
SH	Solihull Hospital Archive
CJ	Taken by the late Cliff Joiner, now part of the above
SL	Solihull Libraries and Arts
Solihull News	Solihull News
EH	Plans drawn by Edna Hale

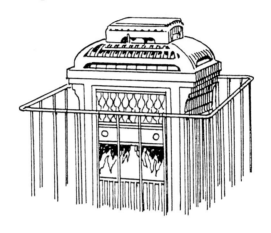